Quick Medical Terminology

Quick Medical Terminology

3rd EDITION

3rd edition by
Shirley Soltesz Steiner, R.N., M.S.
Shirley Soltesz Steiner • Genevieve Love Smith • Phyllis E. Davis

JOHN WILEY & SONS, INC.

New York • Chichester • Brisbane • Toronto • Singapore

Library of Congress Cataloging in Publication Data

Smith, Genevieve Love.
    Quick medical terminology/Genevieve Love Smith,
Phyllis E. Davis, Shirley E. Steiner.—3rd ed.
        p.   cm.—(Wiley self-teaching guides)
    Includes index.
    ISBN 0-471-54267-9
    1. Medicine—Terminology—Programmed instruction.
    I. Davis, Phyllis E. II. Steiner, Shirley E. III. Title. IV. Series.
[DNLM: 1. Nomenclature—programmed instruction. W 15 S648q]
R123.S62   1992
610'.14—dc20
                                                        91-37703

Printed in the United States of America.
10 9

To

Millie Alter, as a small down payment on a
large debt. She cared; therefore this book
exists.

Evelyn Kersten, whose sincere interest and
constant encouragement made a dream
come true.

*Both of these good friends worked much
harder on this manuscript than I had reason
to expect. It's a much better product as a
consequence.*

Burt Steiner, who is my loving husband.

Contents

(*continued on page viii*)

To the Reader

What It Is and Who It's For

Quick Medical Terminology is an easy and enjoyable way of learning to pronounce, spell, and define medical terms used in today's health care settings. You will learn to understand medical terms by breaking them into their component parts, learning the meaning of the parts, and then defining the terms. This word-building strategy will enable you to build a repertoire of medical terms much greater than the 500-plus terms presented in this text.

Learning from this program requires only that you speak and understand the English language and have a high school diploma. That's all you need to begin preparing for a future in one of the nation's fastest growing job markets. This self-teaching guide will help you prepare for a new job or even a new career in the allied health services. You'll learn the very special language of medicine without an instructor. (Although you may be using this program in connection with some class work.)

How to Use This Program

Everything you need for this learning experience is right in your hand. Our self-teaching guide contains not only nine self-instructional units, but also two final tests and a pair of review exercises for each of the units. We suggest using one of the final tests before you start the program and the other after completing all the lessons in the book. Pre- and post-testing will show you how much you have learned.

Numbered frames are the building blocks of each unit. A frame presents a small amount of information and asks you to respond to that information. Your answer usually will involve making a choice, writing a word or a brief definition, labelling an illustration, or matching terms with their definitions. We provide the correct answer for you on the left-hand side of the page. It is a good idea to use a folded piece of paper to cover the answers until you give your answer. Your answer will be correct most of the time. When your answer doesn't match our answer, be sure you understand why not. If you need help, go back and review a few frames before continuing.

This self-teaching guide lets you proceed at a pace that is right for you. That means you may take as much time as you need to complete a unit. Some units are longer than others and you may be unable to finish an entire unit in one sitting. To help you plan your breaks, we designed several short learning sequences into each unit. You'll recognize a learning sequence because it ends with a brief review exercise. If you need a break, stop after a review exercise. After about 1 to 1½ hours of studying, take some time out to relax.

A final exercise in each unit pulls together all the new words introduced in the unit. Here's your opportunity to practice pronouncing each term correctly and defining it aloud or sub-verbally (saying it to yourself). We provide a pronunciation guide alongside each term in the list to help you practice pronouncing it correctly. You might ask a friend to pronounce each term in the list so you can practice spelling it when you hear it.

Be sure to practice what you've already learned. In the back of the book we have provided a two-part review exercise for each of the nine instructional units that make up this program. Review Sheet, Part 1 may be used immediately after completing a unit. This exercise recaps what you just studied. Review Sheet, Part 2 will help you recall terms and definitions of the preceding unit before you begin the next unit. You may use these Review Sheets any time and as often as you wish. We suggest you make several photocopies of each Review Sheet and use them at any time to practice what you've already covered.

Why This Program Does What It Does

Active participation is the key to our word-building strategy. It will set you on the road to an ever-expanding medical vocabulary. You will start by building on what you already know to help you learn what you don't know. You will learn quickly and easily if you carefully read the information presented to you and then actually follow the directions and do what is called for. WRITE your answers. PRONOUNCE the terms. Get involved with your own learning.

PRACTICE, PRACTICE, PRACTICE. This self-teaching guide helps you discover connections and relationships for developing a large reservoir of medical terms. The exercises are new, different, comfortable, and challenging. Diagrams, tables, and illustrations support your learning. We use repetition, practice, and review to help you develop a thorough understanding of useful medical terms. But don't wait until you finish the whole course before practicing what you have studied. Put your words to work as quickly and as often as you can.

Two concerns guided the selection of terms used in this program. First, how useful are these terms for current jobs in the health care industry? And second, how well do they work in the exercises to provide the basis for continuous learning and building of a substantial vocabulary? Our selection includes three basic categories of terms: integral terms, anatomical terms, and compound words. Examples of integral or whole and complete terms include epistaxis, singultus, and ventral. Word roots and combining forms are derived from anatomical terms. For example, the word root for thorax is thorac-, the combining form is thoraco-. For iris, it's ir- and irido-. Compound terms are formed from one or more word roots plus prefixes and suffixes: appendic/itis, en/cephalo/rrhagia, lipo/chondr/oma.

Stedman's Medical Dictionary, 25th Edition, is the reference for all terms and their definitions. However, the editor reworded and simplified many of the definitions to meet program objectives and your needs and background. Some terms do not include all the details or all possible meanings that appear in the reference. Refer to your medical dictionary if you have any questions.

Good learning, and have fun!

S.E.S.

Objectives of the Program

When you have finished *Quick Medical Terminology*, you will have formed over 500 medical terms using the word-building system, combining prefixes, suffixes, word roots, and combining forms.

1. You will learn to understand medical terms by breaking them into their component parts and learning the meaning of the parts.

2. You will be able to apply this strategy to terms covered in this book and others you will come across as you work in a health-care setting.

Pronunciation Key

The primary stress mark (´) is placed after the syllable bearing the heavier stress or accent; the secondary stress mark (´) follows a syllable having a somewhat lighter stress, as in *com·men·da·tion* (kom´ ən·dā´ shən).

a	add, map	m	move, seem	u	up, done
ā	ace, rate	n	nice, tin	er	urn, term
air	care, air	ng	ring, song	yōō	use, few
ä	palm, father	o	odd, hot	v	vain, eve
b	bat, rub	ō	open, so	w	win, away
ch	check, catch	ô	order, jaw	y	yet, yearn
d	dog, rod	oi	oil, boy	z	zest, muse
e	end, pet	ou	out, now	zh	vision, pleasure
ē	even, tree	ōō	pool, food	ə	the schwa, an
f	fit, half	oo	took, full		unstressed vowel
g	go, log	p	pit, stop		representing the
h	hope, hate	r	run, poor		sound spelled
i	it, give	s	see, pass		*a* in *above*
ī	ice, write	sh	sure, rush		*e* in *sicken*
j	joy, ledge	t	talk, sit		*i* in *clarity*
k	cool, take	th	thin, both		*o* in *melon*
l	look, rule	th	this, bathe		*u* in *focus*

Source: Slightly modified "Pronunciation Key" in *Funk & Wagnalls Standard College Dictionary.* Copyright © 1977 by Harper & Row, Publishers, Inc. Reprinted by permission of the publisher.

The schwa (ə) varies widely in quality from a sound close to the (u) in *up* to a sound close to the (i) in *it* as heard in pronunciations of such words as *ballot, custom, landed, horses.*

The (r) in final position as in *star* (stär) and before a consonant as in *heart* (härt) is regularly indicated in the respellings, but pronunciations without (r) are unquestionably reputable. Standard British is much like the speech of Eastern New England and the Lower South in this feature.

In a few words, such as *button* (but′n) and *sudden* (sud′n), no vowel appears in the unstressed syllable because the (n) constitutes the whole syllable.

The Word-Building System

Quick Medical Terminology teaches a system of word building. It has exceptions, of course, but once you have learned the system you will be able to build thousands of words. Medicine has a large vocabulary, but you can learn much of it by following the system and putting words together from their parts.

port

1.
All words have a word root. This is the foundation of a word. The foundation of trans/port, ex/port, im/port, and sup/port is the word root

_____.

word root

2.
Suf/fix, pre/fix, af/fix, and fix/ation have fix as their _____.

tonsill

3.
What is the word root in tonsill/itis, tonsill/ectomy, and tonsill/ar? _____.

word roots

4.
Compound words are formed when two (or more) word roots are used to build the word. Even in ordinary English, compound words are formed from two or more _____.

5.
Sometimes the two word roots are words. They still form a compound word. Is short/hand a compound word? _____. Explain your answer.
_____
_____
_____.

Yes.
It is formed from
   two words: short
   and hand

6.
Form a compound word, using the words under and age: _____.

underage

7.
Form a compound word from the word roots under and nutrition: _____.

undernutrition

8.
A combination of two or more words or two or more word roots means that the word formed is a _____.

compound word

9.
A combining form is word root plus a vowel. In the word therm/o/meter, the combining form is _____/____.

therm/o

10.
In the word speed/o/meter, speed/o is the _____.

combining form

11.
In the compound words micr/o/scope, micr/o/film, and micr/o/be, the word root is _____; the combining form is _____/____.

micr
micr/o

therm/o
meter

12.
Compound words can also be formed from the combining form of the word root and a whole word. In the word therm/o/meter, the combining form is _____/_____; the whole word is _____.

micr/o/film
hydr/o/meter

13.
In each of the following compound words, circle the whole word. Underline just the word root:
micr/o/film
hydr/o/meter

micr/o
scop (or micro)
-ic

14.
In medical terminology, compound words are usually built from a combining form, a word root, and an ending. In the word micr/o/scop/ic, the combining form is _____/___; a word root is _____; the ending is _____.

electr/o/stat/ic

15.
Build a word from the combining form electr/o, the word root stat, the ending -ic:
_____/___/_____/__.

combining form
word root
ending

16.
In the word electr/o/metr/ic,
electr/o is the _____;
metr is the _____;
-ic is the _____.

-er, -ed, -ing

17.
The ending that follows a word root is a suffix. In the words plant/er, plant/ed, plant/ing, the suffixes are _____, _____, _____.

18.
You can change the meaning of a word by adding a suffix. The suffix -er means one who. The word root port means to carry. When you add the suffix -er (port/er), the word means

one who carries

_____.

19.
Able changes the meaning of read in the word read/able; able is a _____.

suffix

20.
A prefix is a word part that goes before a word, or some form of a word, and changes its meaning. In the words im/plant, sup/plant, and trans/plant, the prefixes are _____, _____, _____.

im-, sup-, trans-

21.
In the word dis/please, dis- comes before and changes the meaning of please; dis- is a

prefix

_____.

22.
Before studying more, review what you have learned. The foundation of a word is called the

word root

_____.

23.
A word part placed before a word to change its meaning is a _____.

prefix

24.
A word part that follows a word root and changes its meaning is a _____.

suffix

25.
When a vowel is added to a word root, the word
part resulting is called the _____

combining form   _____.

26.
When some form of two or more word roots
combines to form a word, that word is called a

compound word   _____.

Unit 1

In Unit 1 you will make more than 30 new words by using the following word roots and suffixes:

acr/o (*extremities*)
cardi/o (*heart*)
cyan/o (*blue*)
cyt/o (*cell*)
dermat/o, derm/o (*skin*)
duoden/o (*duodenum*)
electr/o (*electrical*)

eti/o (*cause*)
gastr/o (*stomach*)
gram/o (*record*)
leuk/o (*white*)
megal/o (*enlarged*)
path/o (*disease*)

-algia (*pain*)
-ectomy (*excision of*)
-itis (*inflammation of*)
-ologist (*one who studies, a specialist*)

-ology (*study of*)
-osis (*condition of*)
-ostomy (*forming a new opening*)
-otomy (*incision into*)
-tome (*instrument that cuts*)

acr/o, or acr	**1.** Acr/o means extremities (arms, hands, legs, and feet). To refer to extremities, physicians use words containing _____/____.
acr/o	**2.** Acr/o concerns extremities, which in the human body are also known as limbs. To build words referring to arms, use _____/____.
acr/o	**3.** To build words about the legs, use _____/____.

4.
Acr/o any place in a word should make you think of the extremities. When you read a word containing acr or acr /o, you think of

extremities

_____.

5.
The words acr/o/megal/y (acromegaly), acr/o/cyan/osis (acrocyanosis), and acr/o/dermat/itis (acrodermatitis) all refer to the

extremities

_____.

6.
Megal/o means enlarged or oversized. A word containing megal/o will mean that something is

oversized, big, or
enlarged

_____.

7.
Acr/o/megal/y (acromegaly) means that the extremities are _____.

oversized, or
enlarged

8.
Acr/o/megal/y means enlargement of the extremities. The word that means a person has enlarged hands is _____/___/_____/___.

acr/o/megal/y
acromegaly
ak rō meg´ a lē

9.
Occasionally you see a person with very large hands, feet, nose, and chin. The skin also has a coarse texture. The person probably has

acromegaly

_____/_____.
extremities   enlarged

10.
Dermat/o refers to the skin. A dermat/o/logist (dermatologist) is a specialist in a field of medicine who specializes in diseases of the _____.

skin

11.

acr/o/dermat/itis
acrodermatitis
ak rō der′ ma tī′ tis

Acr/o/dermat/itis (acrodermatitis) is a word that means inflammation of the skin of the extremities. A person with red, inflamed hands has

_____/___/_____/_____.

12.

acrodermatitis

A simpler way to say that a patient is suffering from an inflammation of the hands, lower arms, feet, and legs is to say that the person has

_____.

13.

inflammation of

Remembering that the word acrodermatitis means inflammation of the skin of the extremities, draw a conclusion: -itis is a suffix that means

_____.

14.

cyan or cyan/o

Cyan/o is used in words to mean blue or blueness. Acr/o/cyan/osis means blueness of the extremities. The part of the word that tells you the color blue is involved is _____.

15.

osis
condition

The suffix osis makes the word a noun and means condition. To describe a condition of blueness of the extremities, use the suffix _____.
Acrocyanosis is the abnormal _____ of bluish extremities.

16.

acr/o/cyan/osis
acrocyanosis
ak rō sī ə nō′sis

Acrocyanosis, or blueness of the extremities, is usually related to the amount of oxygen getting to the hands and feet. When the heart doesn't pump enough blood containing oxygen, the patient exhibits _____/___/_____/____.

17.
When the lungs cannot get enough oxygen into the blood because of asthma, blueness of the extremities may result. This is another cause of

acrocyanosis   _____.

18.
blueness
of the extremities   Acrocyanosis means _____
_____.

19.
Dermat/osis denotes an abnormal skin condition.
-osis   The suffix that means condition is _____.

20.
cyan/osis   Osis is a suffix meaning a condition. Build a word
cyanosis   that means a condition of blueness:
sī ə nō´sis   _____ / _____.

21.
dermat/osis
dermatosis   Build a word that means a condition of the skin:
der ma tō´sis   _____ / _____.

22.
The Greek word *tomos* means a piece cut off. From this word we have many combining forms that refer to cutting: ec/tom/y (cut out), o/tom/y (cut into), -tome (an instrument that cuts). A
skin   dermatome is an instrument that cuts _____.

23.
dermat/ome
dermatome   A dermatome is an instrument. When a physician
derm´ə tōm   wants a thin slice of a patient's skin for a skin graft,
the doctor asks for a _____ / _____.

24.

a bluish discolor-
ation of the skin

Derm/o, dermat/o refer to the skin. Cyan/o/derm/a
(cyanoderma) means _____
_____ .

a disease
of the skin

Dermat/osis (dermatosis) means _____
_____ .

25.

cyan/o/derm/a
cyanoderma
sī ə nō der′mä

Cyanoderma sometimes occurs when children
swim too long in cold water. If a patient has a
bluish discoloration of the skin for any reason, the
person suffers from _____/ /_____/____ .

26.

leuk or leuk/o

Leuk/o means white or abnormally white. In the
word leuk/o/derm/a, the part that means white is
_____ .

white skin, or
abnormally
white skin

27.

Leuk/o/derm/a means _____
_____ .

28.

leuk/o/derm/a
leukoderma
lōō kō der′ mä

Some people have much less color in their skin
than is normal. Their skin is white. They have
_____/ /_____/____ .

29.

cyt/o

Cyt/o refers to cells. Cytology is the study of cells.
The part of cyt/o/logy that means cells is
_____/__ .

30.
There are several kinds of cells in blood. One kind is the leuk/o/cyte. A leukocyte is a _____ _____.

white cell

31.
There are several different kinds of cells in the blood. When a physician wants to know how many white cells there are, the doctor asks for a _____ / ___ / _____ / ___ count.

leuk/o/cyt/e
leukocyte
loo´ kō sīt

32.
You have heard of leuk/em/ia, popularly called "blood cancer"; ia is a word ending, and em means blood. A term meaning literally "white blood" is _____ / _____ /ia.

leuk/em/ia
leukemia
loo kē´ mē ə

33.
In the word acr/o/megal/y, the root for extremities is _____ / ___ and the word root for oversized is _____.

acr/o
megal

34.
Cardi/o refers to the heart. Megal/o/card/ia means _____.

oversized heart, or
    enlargement of
    the heart

35.
Megalocardia refers to heart muscle. When any muscle exercises, it gets larger. If the heart muscle has to overexercise, _____ / ___ / _____ / ia will probably occur.

megal/o/card/ia
megalocardia
meg ə lō kär´ dē ä

Upper Gastrointestinal System

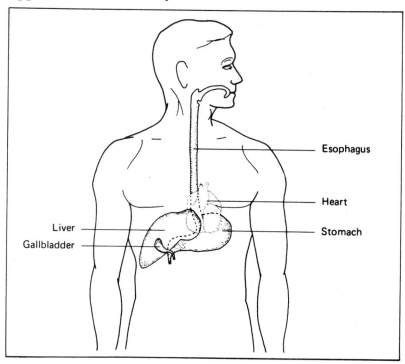

36.

megalocardia

An inadequate supply of oxygen to the heart muscle causes it to beat more often. Inadequate oxygen to the heart may also lead to an enlarged heart, or _____.

37.

megal/o/gastr/ia
megalogastria
meg ə lō gas′ trē ä

Try this one. Gastr is the word root for stomach. When the stomach enlarges so that it crowds other organs, an undesirable condition exists known as
_____ / _____ / _____ / ia .

oversized heart, or
enlargement of
the heart

38.

Megalocardia means _____
_____.

39.

inflammation
of the heart

Cardi/o refers to the heart. Card/itis means

_____.

40.

Here's a quick review. Using the suggested
answers, write the meaning of each of the
following terms.

SUGGESTED ANSWERS:

abnormal condition of	heart
blueness	inflammation of
cell	skin
cutting instrument	stomach
enlarged, oversized	white
extremities	

extremities   acr/o _____.
blueness   cyan/o _____.
white   leuk/o _____.
stomach   gastr/o _____.
cell   cyt/o _____.
heart   cardi/o _____.
enlarged, oversized   megal/o _____.
skin   derm/o, dermat/o _____.
abnormal condition of -osis _____.
inflammation of   -itis _____.
cutting instrument   -tome _____.

41.

Now build a medical term for each of the following:

megalo/card/ia   enlarged heart: _____/ _____/ ia.

acro/megal/y   oversized extremities: _____/ _____ /y.
                                          extremities   oversized

leuko/cyt/e   white cell: _____/ _____/e.
                               white   cell

dermat/itis   inflammation of the skin: _____/ _____.

42.
Let's have a change of pace here. Professional health workers use some special words to talk about illness and sick people. Here are just a few you'll find very useful. Read each definition. Then underline a key word or two to help you remember what the term means.

It's up to you, of course, but here are some key words.

sickness, illness

Disease is a condition in which bodily health is impaired. It means sickness or illness.

exhibition, display, evidence

Manifestation is proof of impaired bodily health. It's a display, exhibition, or evidence of disease.

changes (structural and functional)

Pathology is the scientific study of changes in the human body (structural and functional) caused by disease.

causes

Etiology is the scientific study of causes of disease.

You may refer to the definitions if you need help answering frames 43 to 48.

The cause of the patient's disease is not yet known (and may remain unknown).

43.
If a physician says that a patient's disease is of unknown etiology, what would that mean to you?

_____

_____

44.
sickness, illness   Another word for disease is _____.

45.
evidence   Manifestation is a display, or _____, of disease.

46.

causes

Etiology is the scientific study of _____ of disease.

47.

changes

Pathology is the study of _____ caused by disease.

48.

Select the best term for each definition. Write your choice in the space provided.

pathology   etiology   manifestation   disease

disease

Another term for illness or sickness is _____.

manifestation

Evidence, or proof, of disease is _____.

etiology

The study of causes of disease is _____.

pathology

The scientific study of changes caused by disease is _____.

49.

The combining forms logy and logist are suffixes you will use for convenience.
log/y—means the study of,
log/ist—means one who studies.
One who studies changes caused by disease is a

path/o/logist

path / __ / _____.

50.

cardi/o/logist
cardiologist
kär dē ol´ ə jist

A cardiologist diagnoses heart disease. The specialist who determines that a heart is deformed is a _____ / __ / _____.
              heart   specialist

cardiologist

51.
A physician who reads electr/o/cardi/o/grams (records of electrical impulses given off by the heart) is also a _____.

a record of
  electrical waves
  given off by the
  heart (or
  equivalent)

52.
Give the meaning of electr/o/cardi/o/gram.
(Gram/o is a combining form that means record.)

_____

_____.

electr/o/cardi/o/
  gram
electrocardiogram
ē lek′ trō kär′ dē ə
  gram

53.
The electr/o/cardi/o/gram is a record obtained by electr/o/cardi/o/graph/y. A technician can learn electrocardiography, but it takes a cardiologist to read the

_____/____/_____/____/_____.
electrical   heart   record

54.
A physician can take a chart that looks like this,

cardiologist
electrocardiogram

and learn something about a person's heart. That kind of physician is a _____ and is reading an _____.

cardi/algia
cardialgia
kär dē al′ jē a

55.
The suffix algia means pain. Form a word that means heart pain: _____/_____.
                                heart   pain

cardialgia

56.
When a patient complains of pain in the heart, the symptom is known medically as

_____.

57.

stomach
-algia

Gastralgia means pain in the stomach. Gastr/o
means _____. The suffix for pain is

_____.

58.

stomach
excision or removal

Gastr/ectomy means excision (removal) of all or
part of the stomach. Gastr/o means _____.
Ectomy means _____.

59.

gastr/ectomy
gastrectomy
gas trek´ tō mē

A gastr/ectomy is a surgical procedure. When a
stomach ulcer has perforated, a partial
_____/_____ may be indicated.
stomach   excision of

60.

gastrectomy

Cancer of the stomach may require a surgeon to
remove all or part of the patient's stomach. This
procedure is a _____.

61.

gastr/itis
gastritis
gas trī´ tis

Form a word that means inflammation of the
stomach. _____/_____.

62.

duoden/um
duodenum
dōō ōd´ nəm (or
  dōō ō dē´ nəm)

The duoden/um is the part of the small intestine
that connects with the stomach. Duoden/o refers to
the _____/_____.

63.

forming a new
  opening
  between the
  stomach and
  duodenum

The suffix -ostomy means forming a new opening.
Gastr/o/duoden/ostomy means _____

_____.

gastr/o/duoden/
   ostomy
gastroduoden-
   ostomy
gas´ trō dōō ō de
   nos´ tō mē

64.
A surgeon who removes the natural connection between the duodenum and stomach and then forms a new connection is doing a

_____ / / _____ / _____.

65.
A gastroduodenostomy is a surgical procedure. When the pyloric sphincter, a valve that controls the amount of food going from the stomach to the duodenum, no longer functions, a

gastroduoden-
   ostomy

_____ may be done.

66.
The suffix -ectomy means excision of; -ostomy means forming a new opening. The form -o/tom/y means incision into. A duo/den/otomy is an

duodenum

incision into the _____.

67.

-otomy

The suffix for incision into is _____.

duoden/otomy
duodenotomy
dōō od ə not´ ə mē

If a physician makes an incision into the wall of the duodenum, the doctor has performed a

_____ / _____.

68.

-itis

The suffix for inflammation is _____.

duoden/itis
duodenitis
dōō od ə nī´ tis

The word for inflammation of the duodenum is

_____ / _____.

69.

of, or pertaining to,
mother; of, or
pertaining to,
father

Duoden/al means of, or pertaining to, the
duodenum; -al is an ending that means of, or
pertaining to. Matern/al means _____.
patern/al means _____.

70.

duoden/al
duodenal
do͞o ō dē´ nəl

In the sentence "Duodenal carcinoma was
present," the word meaning of, or pertaining to,
the duodenum is _____/____.

71.

duoden/ostomy
duodenostomy
do͞o od ə nos´ tō
mē

The suffix -ostomy means making a new opening.
The word to form a new opening into the
duodenum is _____/_____.

72.

gastroduoden-
ostomy

Here's one for you to figure out. A duodenostomy
can be formed in more than one manner. If it is
formed with the stomach, it is called a

_____.

stomach   duodenum   new opening

73.

-ostomy

The suffix for forming a new opening is

_____.

74.

Let's review what you've covered. Using the
suggested answers, write the meaning of each of
the following terms.

SUGGESTED ANSWERS:

blueness	duodenum
cell	electrical
causes	enlarged, oversized
changes due to disease	record of

duodenum   duoden/o _____.
changes due to disease   path/o _____.

record of	gram/o _____.
cell	cyt/o _____.
electrical	electr/o _____.
causes	eti/o _____.
enlarged, oversized	megal/o _____.
blueness	cyan/o _____.

75.
Now try it with the suffixes you just learned.

SUGGESTED ANSWERS:

(abnormal) condition	incision into
cutting instrument	inflammation of
form a new opening	of, or pertaining to
one who studies	pain

of, or pertaining to	-al _____.
inflammation of	-itis _____.
(abnormal) condition	-osis _____.
form a new opening	-ostomy _____.
cutting instrument	-tome _____.
incision into	-otomy _____.
pain	-algia _____.
one who studies	-ologist _____.

76.
Now build some new words.

cyan/osis   A condition of blueness is _____/ _____.
                                                  blueness   condition

One who studies disease changes is a

path/ologist   _____ /_____.
                disease/changes   one who studies

A surgical procedure that makes a new opening in the duodenum is a

duoden/ostomy   _____/ _____.
                duodenum   form a new opening

A term meaning of, or pertaining to, the study of causes of disease is

eti/ologic/al   _____/ /_____/_____.
            causes of disease   the study of   pertaining to

77.

While working through Unit 1, you formed the following new medical terms. Read them one at a time and pronounce each aloud several times until you can articulate each term clearly and correctly.

acrocyanosis (ak rō sī ə nō´ sis)

acrodermatitis (ak rō der´ ma tī´ tis)

acromegaly (ak rō meg´ a lē)

cardialgia (kär dē al´ jē a)

cardiologist (kär dē ol´ ə jist)

carditis (kär dī´ tis)

cyanoderma (sī ə nō der´ mä)

cyanosis (sī ə nō´ sis)

cytology (sī tol´ ə jē)

dermatologist (der ma tol´ ə jist)

dermatome (derm´ ə tōm)

dermatosis (der ma tō´ sis)

disease (diz ēz´)

duodenal (doo ō dē´ nəl)

etiological (ē´ tē ō loj´ i kəl)

gastralgia (gas tral´ jē a)

gastrectomy (gas trek´ tō mē)

gastritis (gas trī´ tis)

gastroduodenostomy (gas´ trō doo ō de nos´ tō mē)

leukemia (loo kē´ mē ə)

leukocyte (loo´ kō sīt)

leukoderma (loo kō der´ mä)

manifestation (man´ ə fes tā´ shən)

megalocardia (meg ə lō kär´ dē ä)

megalogastria (meg ə lō gas´ trē ä)

pathologist (path ol´ ə jist)

pathology (path ol´ ə jē)

Before going on to Unit 2, take the Unit 1 Self-Test.

Unit 1 Self-Test

PART 1

From the list on the right select the correct meaning for each of the following terms. Write the letter in the space provided.

_____ 1. Megalocardia
_____ 2. Duodenostomy
_____ 3. Dermatologist
_____ 4. Gastritis
_____ 5. Electrocardiography
_____ 6. Gastralgia
_____ 7. Pathologist
_____ 8. Acrocyanosis
_____ 9. Etiology
_____ 10. Manifestation

a. Study of, or pertaining to, causes (of disease)
b. A specialist in the field of skin diseases
c. A condition of blueness of the extremities
d. Enlargement of the heart
e. Forming a new opening in the duodenum
f. Display, evidence of disease
g. One who specializes in the study of disease changes
h. Pain in the stomach
i. Inflammation of the stomach
j. Recordings of electrical waves of the heart

PART 2

Write a medical term for each of the following:

1. Impaired bodily health   _____
2. Bluish discoloration of the skin _____
3. White cell   _____
4. Oversized or enlarged stomach   _____
5. Evidence of disease   _____
6. The study of causes of an illness _____
7. Excision or removal of the stomach _____
8. Pertaining to the duodenum   _____
9. Generalized condition of blueness _____
10. Heart pain   _____

ANSWERS

Part 1	Part 2
1. d	1. disease
2. e	2. cyanoderma
3. b	3. leukocyte
4. i	4. megalogastria
5. j	5. manifestation
6. h	6. etiology
7. g	7. gastrectomy
8. c	8. duodenal
9. a	9. cyanosis
10. f	10. cardialgia

Unit 2

In Unit 2 you will put together more than 30 new words, using the following word roots, prefixes, and suffixes.

aden/o (*gland*)
arthr/o (*joint*)
carcin/o (*malignancy*)
cele/o, o/cele (*hernia*)
cephal/o (*head*)
chondr/o (*cartilage*)
cost/o (*ribs*)
dent/o (*tooth*)
emes/is *(vomiting)*
hist/o *(tissue)*

laryng/o (*larynx*)
lip/o *(fat)*
malac/o *(soft)*
morph/o *(structure* of)
muc/o *(mucus)*
onc/o *(tumor)*
ost/o, oste/o *(bone)*
plast/o *(repair)*
troph/o *(development)*

en-, endo- (*in, inside, within*)
ex-, ex/o- (*outside, out*)
hyper- *(excessive)*
hypo- *(under)*
inter- *(between)*

-ia, -ic *(pertaining to)*
-oid *(resembling)*
-oma *(tumor)*

1.

prefix

A prefix goes before a word to change its meaning. In the words hyper/trophy, hyper/emia, and hyper/emesis, the meaning of trophy, emia, and emesis is changed by hyper-. Hyper- means more than normal, an excessive amount. Hyper- is a _____ (prefix/suffix).

2.

hyper-

Hyper/thyroid/ism means overactivity of the thyroid gland. The prefix that expresses higher than normal activity of the thyroid gland is _____.

3.

hyper/emesis
hyperemesis
hī per em´ ə sis

Emesis is a word that means vomiting. A word that means excessive vomiting is

_____/_____.

4.

hyperemesis

Gallbladder attacks can cause excessive vomiting. This, too, is called _____.

5.

hyper/troph/y
hypertrophy
hī per´ trō fē

Hyper/trophy means overdevelopment; troph/o comes from the Greek word for nourishment. Note the connection between nourishment and development. Overdevelopment is called

_____/_____/y.

6.

hypertrophy

Muscles also can overdevelop or

_____.

7.

hypertrophy

Many organs can overdevelop. If the heart overdevelops, the condition is called _____ of the heart.

8.

hypo-

The prefix hypo- is just the opposite of hyper-. The prefix for under or less than normal is

_____.

9.

skin

skin

Derm/o refers to the _____. The suffix -ic means of, or pertaining to. Hypo/derm/ic means under the _____.

10.

hypo/der/mic
hypodermic
hī pō der´ mik

A hypodermic needle is short because it goes just under the skin. A shot that can be given superficially is administered with a

_____ / _____ / _____ needle.
under   skin   pertaining to

11.

aden/itis
adenitis
ad ə nī´ tis

Aden/o is used in words that refer to glands. Build a word that means inflammation of a gland:

_____ / _____.
gland   inflammation of

12.

aden/ectomy
adenectomy
ad ə nek´ tō mē

Since ectomy means excision (or surgical removal of), the word for surgical removal of a gland is

_____ / _____.
gland   surgical removal

13.

adenectomy

If a gland is like a tumor, part or all of it may be excised. Excision of a gland is

_____.

14.

aden/oma
adenoma
ad ə nō´ mä

The suffix for tumor is -oma. Form a word that means tumor of a gland:

_____ / _____.

15.

surgical removal,
 or excision, of
 the thyroid
 gland

Try this. Sometimes the thyroid gland develops a tumor. A patient's history might read, ". . . because of the presence of a thyroid adenoma, thyroidectomy is indicated." What is a thyroid/ectomy? _____

_____

_____.

16.
An adenoma is a glandular tumor; -oma means

tumor
fat, fatty tissue

_____. A lip/oma is a tumor of fatty tissue.
Lip /o is the word root for _____.

lip/oma
lipoma
li pō´ mä

17.
A fatty tumor is called a

_____ / _____.

cancerous tumor

18.
Carcin/o is the root for cancer. A carcin/oma is a
_____.

19.
A carcinoma may occur in almost any part of the
body. Where is a gastric carcinoma located?

in the stomach

_____.

carcinoma
kär sin ō´ mä
carcinoma
duodenal
   carcinoma

20.
A cancerous tumor of the spleen is called splenic
_____. Cancer of the tonsil is
tonsillar _____. Cancer of the
duodenum is _____
_____.

lip/oid
lipoid
lip´ oid

21.
Lipoma is a fatty tumor; -oid is a suffix meaning
like or resembling. Build a word that means fatlike,
or resembling fat: _____.

lipoid

22.
The word lipoid is used in chemistry and pathology. It describes a substance that looks like fat, dissolves like fat, but is not fat. Cholesterol is an alcohol that resembles fat; therefore, cholesterol is _____/_____ .
     fat   like

muc/oid
mucoid
my o͞o´ koid

23.
Muc/oid means resembling mucus. There is a substance in connective tissue that resembles mucus. This is a _____/_____ substance.

resembling mucus

24.
There is a protein in the body that is said to be mucoid in nature. Mucoid means
_____
_____ .

mucoid

25.
A substance that resembles mucus is said to be _____ .

laryng/itis
laryngitis
lair an jī´ tis

26.
The larynx contains the vocal cords. Laryng/o builds words that refer to the larynx. Form a word that means inflammation of the larynx:
_____/_____ .
 larynx   inflammation of

inflammation
    of the larynx

27.
After a bad cold a patient may develop laryngitis, which means _____
_____ .

28.

An obstruction of the colon may require a new opening into the colon that will be *permanent*.

Col/, col/o refers to the colon, or large bowel. The suffix -ostomy means a new (permanent) opening into.

(kō los′ tō mē)
a new opening
  (permanent)
  into the colon

Col/ostomy means _____

_____.

29.

The suffix for a new (permanent) opening is

-ostomy

_____.

30.

An obstruction of the windpipe makes breathing very difficult, or even impossible. In an emergency, a physician may make an incision into the windpipe to permit a free flow of air to the patient's lungs.

Trache, trache/o refers to the trachea, or windpipe. The suffix -otomy means incision into, or a *temporary* opening.

(trā kē ot′ ō mē)
an incision into,
  or temporary
  opening into,
  the trachea

Trache/otomy means _____

_____.

31.

The suffix meaning a temporary opening, or

-otomy

incision into, is _____.

32.

Which suffix would you use to indicate creation of

-ostomy

a new (permanent) opening? _____.

Which suffix means making an incision into, or

-otomy

creating a temporary opening? _____.

creation of a new
   (permanent)
   opening into
   the colon

33.
Colostomy means

_____.

incision into, or
   temporary
   opening into,
   the trachea

Tracheotomy means

_____.

34.
Time for a quick review. Using the suggested
answers, write a meaning for each of the following
word roots.

SUGGESTED ANSWERS:

fat, fatty	mucus
larynx	skin
cancer, malignant	spleen

fat, fatty   lip/o _____.
spleen   splen/o _____.
skin   derm/o _____.
larynx   laryng/o _____.
mucus   muc/o _____.
cancer, malignant   carcin/o _____.

35.
Now do the same with the following suffixes.

SUGGESTED ANSWERS:

incision into, temporary opening	a new (permanent) opening into
like, or resembling	development
of, or pertaining to	vomiting
tumor	excision of

development   -trophy _____.
excision of   -ectomy _____.

incision into,
   temporary
   opening   -otomy _____.
a new (permanent)
   opening into   -ostomy _____.
of, or pertaining to -ic, -ar, -al _____.
like, or resembling   -oid _____.
vomiting   -emesis _____.
tumor   -oma _____.

36.
Complete the following:

under, less   Hypo- is a prefix meaning _____.

over, excessive Hyper- is a prefix meaning _____.

37.
Build a medical term for each of the following:

muc/oid   resembling mucus _____/_____.
                                    mucus   like

splen/ic   pertaining to the spleen _____/_____.
                                            spleen   of the

aden/ectomy   excision of a gland _____/_____.
                                       gland   excision of

hyper/trophy   overdevelopment _____/_____.
                                   excessive   development

hypo/derm/ic   under the skin _____/_____/_____.
                                  under   skin   pertaining to

laryng/ostomy   new (permanent) opening into the larynx
                 _____/_____.
                 larynx   new opening

38.
At this stage of word building, students sometimes
find that they have one big headache. The word for
pain in the head is cephal/algia. The word root for
cephal   head is _____.

The Head

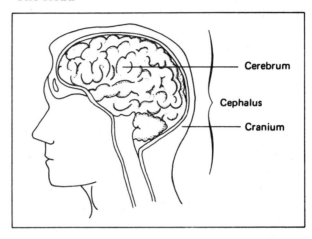

Cerebrum

Cephalus

Cranium

Use this illustration to help you with frames
38 to 47.

39.

cephal/algia
cephalalgia
(sef ə lal´ jē ä)

If you are now suffering from a headache,
persevere, for later this gets to be fun. Any pain in
the head may be called

_____/_____.
head   pain

40.

cephalalgia

The word root for head is cephal/o. The word for
pain in the head is _____.

41.

headache

Cephalalgia means _____.

42.

pertaining
to the head

Cephal/ic means _____
_____.

43.

cephal/ic
cephalic
sə fal′ ik

A case history reporting head wounds due to an accident might read, "_____ / _____ lacerations present."

44.

cephalic

A tumor located on the head might be noted as a _____ tumor.

PREFIX	MEANING
en-, endo-	in, inside, within
ex-, exo-	out, outside completely

Use the table to help with frames 45 to 52.

45.

inside the head,
  the brain

Cephal/o means head. What does encephal/o mean? _____.

46.

brain

Since the brain is enclosed inside the head's bony vault, encephal/o means the organ inside the head, or the _____.

47.

encephalitis
en sef ə lī′ tis

Build words meaning the following:
inflammation of the brain
_____ / _____.
brain   inflammation of

encephaloma
en sef′ ə lō′ mä

brain tumor _____ / _____.
                    brain   tumor of

48.

inflammation
  within the heart

What does endocarditis mean? _____
_____.

49.
A prefix meaning out, or completely outside, of is

ex-, or exo-

_____.

50.
Exo/genous means originating completely outside of an organ or part. Genous takes its meaning from a Latin word meaning to produce or originate. What part of the term means completely outside

exo-

of? _____.

Exogenous refers to something that originates completely outside of an organism, cell, or organ. Build a word that indicates something is

endo/genous
en´ doj´ ə nus

produced or originates from within a cell or organism: _____/_____.
                                within   produced or originating

51.
Try these. Here are some common English words often used in the medical world. Write what each means.
hale (breathe)   cise (cut)   spire (breathe)

breathe out

cut out

breathe out (it also
   means to die or
   breathe out for the
   last time)

exhale means _____.

excise means _____.

expire means _____.

52.
Write two forms of a prefix for each of the following.

en-, endo-
ex-, exo-

in, inside of, within _____, _____.
out, completely outside of _____, _____.

53.
The Greek word for hernia is *kele*. From this we derive the combining forms cele/o or o/cele. Encephal/o/cele is a word meaning herniation of

brain

_____ tissue.

54.

encephal/o/cele
encephalocele
en səf´ a lō sēl

Any hernia is a protrusion of a part from its natural cavity. Herniation is expressed by cele. A protrusion of brain tissue from its natural cavity is

an _____ / ___ / _____.
       brain   hernia

55.

encephalocele

Increased fluid inside the head sometimes causes herniation. Herniation of the brain in medical language is called an _____.

56.

softened brain
   tissue

Malac/ia is a word meaning soft, or softened, tissue. Encephal/o/malac/ia means _____

_____.

encephal/o/
   malac/ia
encephalomalacia
en sef´ a lō mä
   la´ zhə

57.
Malac/o is the word root. Softened brain tissue is

_____ / ___ / _____ / ia .
brain   softened

58.
An accident that causes brain injury could result in softened brain tissue called

encephalomalacia

_____.

59.
Oste/o is the root referring to bone. A word
meaning inflammation of the bone is

_____.

oste/itis
osteitis
os tē ī´ tis

60.
What do you think oste/o/malac/ia means?

_____.

soft bones

61.
When calcium leaves the bones and they lose some
of their hardness, the disorder is called

_____ / ___ / _____ / ia .
bone   softened

oste/o/malac/ia
osteomalacia
os´ tē ō mä lā´ zhə

62.
A disorder of the parathyroid gland can cause
calcium to be withdrawn from the bones. When
this occurs, _____ results.

osteomalacia

63.
A hard outgrowth on any bone could be a bone
tumor. In medical terms, it would be referred to as
an _____ / _____.

oste/oma
osteoma
os tē ō´ mä

What does endosteoma mean?

_____.

a tumor inside
(the center
canal of the
bone)

64.
Arthr/o refers to joints; plast/y means surgical
repair of. What does arthr/o/plast/y mean?

_____.

surgical repair of a
joint

65.

Think of a plast/ic surgeon building a new nose or doing a face lift. These are surgical repairs. When a joint has lost its ability to move, movement can sometimes be restored by an

arthr/o/plast/y
arthroplasty
arth´ rō plas´ tē

_____ / _____ / _____ / y.
joint   repair of

66.

If a child is born without a joint, sometimes one can be formed by a surgical procedure called

arthroplasty

_____ .

67.

Form a word that means inflammation of a joint:

arthr/itis
arthritis
ärth rī´ tis

_____ / _____ .
joint   inflammation of

68.

Now form a word that means incision into a joint:

arthr/otomy
arthrotomy
ärth rot´ ō mē

_____ / _____ .
joint   temporary opening

69.

The word oste/o/chondr/itis means inflammation of the bone and cartilage. The word root for cartilage must be _____ / .

chondr/o

70.

Analyze oste/o/chondr/itis:

oste/o
chondr
-itis

_____ combining form for bone,
_____ word root for cartilage,
_____ suffix for inflammation.

oste/o/chondr/itis
osteochondritis
os´ tē ō kon drī´ tis

71.
Now put all the parts together:
_____ / / _____ / _____.
bone   cartilage   inflammation of

inflammation of
  bone and
  cartilage

What does it mean? _____
_____.

excision
  of cartilage

72.
Chondr/ectomy means _____
_____.

inter-

73.
Cost/al means pertaining to the ribs. Inter/cost/al
means between the ribs. The prefix for between is
_____.

inter/cost/al
intercostal
in ter kos´ t'l

74.
There are short strong muscles between the ribs.
These muscles move the ribs during breathing and
are called _____ / _____ / al muscles.
             between   ribs

intercostal

75.
One set of between-the-ribs muscles enlarges the
rib cage when breathing in. When exhaling, the rib
cage is made smaller by another set of
_____ muscles.
(between-the-ribs)

teeth
teeth

spaces between
  the teeth

76.
A dent/ist takes care of _____. A dent/ifrice
is used for cleaning _____.
Interdental spaces means
_____
_____.

dent/algia
dentalgia
den tal´ jē a

77.
Try making a few new words. Pain in the teeth, or
a toothache, is called _____ / _____.

dent/oid
dentoid
den´ toid

A word that means tooth-shaped or resembling a
tooth is _____ / _____.

78.
Try these. Pathogenic means something that
produces disease.

(If you're not sure,
use your
dictionary.)

What is a pathogenic organism? _____
What does pathology mean? _____
Therefore, pathological means _____
_____.

79.
Explain each of the following statements in simple
language.
Hyperemesis is a manifestation of a pathological
condition.
_____

Encephalography is almost always the first step
toward a diagnosis of encephalopathy.
_____

80.
It's time to review again. Using the suggested
answers, write the meaning of each of the
following terms.

SUGGESTED ANSWERS:

bone	joint
cartilage	rib
head	soft, soften
hernia	tooth, teeth

joint
hernia
head

arthr/o _____.
cele/o _____.
cephal/o _____.

cartilage   chondr/o _____.
rib   cost/o _____.
tooth, teeth   dent/o _____.
soft, soften   malac/o_____.
bone   ost/o, oste/o_____.

repair of   **81.**
  (restoration or   These word parts are used as suffixes.
  plastic surgery)   -plasty means _____.
hernia   -cele means _____.

                     82.
in, within, inside   These are easy.
out, completely   end-, endo- is a prefix meaning _____.
  outside of   ex-, exo- is a prefix meaning _____.

                     83.
                     Build a medical term for each of the following.
arthro/plasty   restoration of a joint _____/_____.
                                            joint   plastic surgery of
inter/costal   between the ribs _____/_____.
                                        between   ribs
chondro/malacia   softening of cartilage _____/_____.
                                            cartilage   softened
oste/oma   bony tumor _____/_____.
                                  bone   tumor of
encephalo/cele   herniation of the brain _____/_____.
                                             inside the head   hernia of
dent/oid   resembling teeth _____/_____.
                                        teeth   resembling

84.
You just learned the suffix -oma, meaning tumor. Now, here are three more very useful terms that relate to tumors.

Here are our suggestions:

Read each definition. Then underline a key word or two to help you remember what the term means.

tumors

Oncology is the branch of medicine dealing with tumors.

structure

Morphology is the biological science dealing with the structure of an organism or part.

microscopic tissues

Histology is the study of the microscopic tissues that make up a part or a structure.

changes

Pathology is the study of changes in structure and function caused by disease.

85.
Complete each of the following statements. Look back at the definition if necessary.

tumors

Onc/o refers to _____.

tissues

Hist/o refers to _____.

changes

Path/o refers to _____.

structure

Morph/o refers to _____.

86.
Complete each definition.

structure

Morphology is the study of the _____ of an organism.

tissues

Histology is the study of microscopic _____ making up a part or structure.

tumors

Oncology is the study of _____.

changes

Pathology is the study of _____ caused by disease.

87.

Complete each of the following definitions:

One who studies the tissue structure under a

histologist   microscope is a _____.

A specialist in the care and treatment of patients

oncologist   with tumors is an _____.

One who studies the structure of living organisms

morphologist   is a _____.

A specialist who studies changes in structure and

pathologist   function caused by disease is a _____.

88.

Here are more than 30 medical terms you worked with in Unit 2. Read
each one. Review its meaning and pronounce it aloud several times.

adenectomy (ad ə nek´ tō mē)   histology (his tol´ ō jē)
adenitis (ad ə nī´ tis)   hyperemesis (hī per em´ ə sis)
adenoma (ad ə nō´ mä)   hypertrophy (hī per´ tro fē)
arthroplasty (ärth´ rō plas´ tē)   hypodermic (hī pō der´ mik)
arthrotomy (ärth rot´ ō mē)   intercostal (in ter kos´ t'l)
carcinoma (kär sin ō´ mä)   laryngitis (lair an jī´ tis)
cephalalgia (sef ə lal´ jē ä)   lipoid (lip´ oid)
cephalic (se fal´ ik)   lipoma (lī pō´ mä)
chondritis (kon drī´ tis)   morphology (mor fäl´ ō jē)
colostomy (kō los´ tō mē)   mucoid (myoo´ koid)
dentalgia (den tal´ jē ä)   oncology (on kol´ ō jē)
encephalitis (en sef ə lī´ tis)   osteitis (os tē ī´ tis)
encephalocele (en sef´ ə lō sēl)   osteomalacia (os´ tē ō mä lä´ zhə)
encephaloma (en sef´ ə lō´ mä)   pathologist (path ol´ ō jist)
endosteoma (en dos tē ō´ mä)   thyroidectomy (thī roy dek´ tō mē)
exogenous (eks oj´ ə nus)   tracheotomy (trä kē ot´ ō mē)

Before going on to Unit 3, take the Unit 2 Self-Test.

Unit 2 Self-Test

PART 1

From the list on the right, select the correct meaning for each of the following terms. Write the letters in the space provided.

____ 1. Osteomalacia	a. Overdevelopment
____ 2. Adenoma	b. Study of microscopic tissues
____ 3. Intercostal	c. Surgical removal of cartilage
____ 4. Laryngotomy	d. Between the ribs
____ 5. Cephalalgia	e. Surgical repair of a joint
____ 6. Chondrectomy	f. Softening of bone tissue
____ 7. Encephalocele	g. Herniation of brain tissue
____ 8. Hypertrophy	h. Tumor of glandular tissue
____ 9. Arthroplasty	i. Headache
____10. Histology	j. Incision into the larynx

PART 2

Complete each of the medical terms on the right with the appropriate prefix and/or suffix:

1. Surgical removal of the
   thyroid gland   Thyroid _____
2. Inflammation of glandular tissue   Aden _____
3. Malignant tumor   Carcin _____
4. Excessive vomiting   _____ emesis
5. Resembling mucus   Muc _____
6. Tumor specialist   Onc _____
7. Making a new permanent
   opening into the colon   Col _____
8. Inflammation inside the head   _____ cephal _____
9. Tumor of fat tissue   _____ oma
10. Pertaining to the teeth   Dent _____

ANSWERS

Part 1	Part 2
1. f	1. Thyroidectomy
2. h	2. Adenitis
3. d	3. Carcinoma
4. j	4. Hyperemesis
5. i	5. Mucoid
6. c	6. Oncologist
7. g	7. Colostomy
8. a	8. Encephalitis
9. e	9. Lipoma
10. b	10. Dental

Unit 3

In Unit 3 you will put together at least 50 new words, using the following word roots, prefixes, and suffixes.

abdomin/o (*abdomen*)
cerebr/o (*cerebrum*)
chol/e (*bile, gall*)
cocc/i (*coccus*)
crani/o (*cranium*)
cyst/o (*bladder, sac*)
dipl/o (*double*)
hydr/o (*water*)
lith/o (*stone, calculus*)
lumb/o (*loin*)

metr/o, meter (*measure*)
ot/o (*ear*)
pelv/i (*pelvis*)
phob/ia (*fear*)
py/o (*pus*)
rhin/o (*nose*)
staphyl/o (*grape*)
strept/o (*chain*)
therap/o (*treatment*)
thorac/o (*thorax*)

ab- (*away from*)
ad- (*toward*)
supra- (*above*)

-ar (*pertaining to*)
-centesis (*puncture*)
-genesis, gen/o (*produce, originate*)
-meter (*measuring instrument*)
-orrhea (*flow, discharge*)

1.
The prefix ab- means from or away from.

away from   Abnormal means _____ normal.

2.
The prefix ab- means _____

from or away from   _____.

wandering from
   (the normal
   course of
   events)

3.
Ab/errant uses the prefix ab- before the English word for wandering. Ab/errant means

_____.

ab/errant
aberrant
ab er´ ant

4.
Ab/errant is used in medicine to describe a structure that wanders from the normal. When some nerve fibers follow an unusual route, they form an _____/_____ nerve.

aberrant

5.
Aberrant nerves wander from the normal nerve track. Blood vessels that follow an unusual path are called _____ vessels.

ab/duct/ion
abduction
ab duk´ shun

6.
Ab/duct/ion means movement away from a midline. When the hand is raised from the side of the body, _____/_____/_____ has occurred.

abducted

7.
When children have been kidnapped and taken from their parents, they have been _____.

abducted

8.
Abduction can occur from any midline. When the fingers of the hand are spread apart, four fingers have been _____.

ad/duction
adduction
ad duk´ shun

9.
On the other hand, ad- is a prefix meaning toward. Movement toward a midline is

_____/_____.

10.

ab-

ad-

The prefix meaning from or away from is _____.
The prefixing meaning toward, or toward the midline, is _____.

11.

ad/<u>hesion</u>

When two normally separate tissues join together, they adhere to each other like adhesive tape. Underline the part of the word that means sticking or joining: ad/hesion.

12.

ad/hesion
adhesion
ad hē´ zhun

Several years ago patients did not walk soon enough after surgery, which sometimes resulted in abnormal joining of tissues to each other. Write the word that means the abnormal joining and healing together of tissues: _____/_____.

Abdomen, Cranium, Pelvis & Thorax

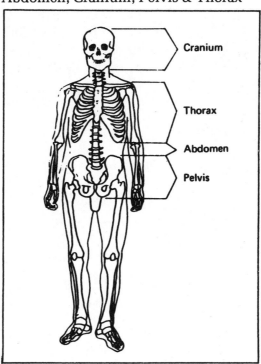

13.
Now patients walk the day following an
appendectomy. This has nearly eliminated

adhesions

_____.

Refer to the illustration on page 47 to help you
complete Frames 14 through 51.

14.
Abdomin/o is used to form words about the
abdomen. When you see abdomin/o in a word, you

abdomen
ab dō´ men

think of the _____.

15.

pertaining to the
abdomen

Abdomin/al is an adjective that means

_____.

16.

abdomin/o/
centesis
abdominocentesis
ab dom´ i nō sen
tē´ sis

Abdomin/o/centesis means tapping or puncturing
the abdomen to remove fluid. This is a surgical
puncture of a cavity. The word for surgical
puncture of the abdominal cavity is

_____ / _____ / _____.
abdomen   puncture of

17.
Centesis (surgical puncture) of a cavity is a word in
itself. Build a word meaning surgical puncture or
tapping of the abdomen:

abdominocentesis

_____.

18.
When fluid has accumulated in the abdominal
cavity, it can be drained off by an

abdominocentesis

_____.

cardi/o/centesis
cardiocentesis
kär´ dē ō sen tē´
    sis

19.
Try this. The word for surgical puncture of a heart
chamber is _____/_/_____.
              heart   puncture of

cyst

20.
Abdomin/o/cyst/ic means pertaining to the
abdomen and urinary bladder. The word root for
bladder is _____.

bladder

21.
Cyst/o is used to form words that refer to the
_____.

cyst/o

22.
To refer to the urinary bladder or any sac
containing fluid, use some form of
_____/_____.

cyst/otomy
cystotomy

23.
The word for incision into a bladder is
_____/_____.
bladder   incision into

cyst/itis
cystitis

Inflammation of a bladder is
_____.

cyst/ectomy
cystectomy

The word for excision of a bladder is
_____.

24.

Chances are good that by now you have figured out how word parts go together to create meaning. But let's review a simple rule and some examples.

Rule: About 90 percent of the time, the meaning of a term can be unscrambled by identifying its component parts in reverse.

For example,
   cyst means bladder;
   -itis means inflammation of.

inflammation of the bladder

Therefore *cyst/itis* means

_____.

one who studies the skin, or a skin specialist

   Dermat means skin;
   -ologist means a specialist (one who studies).
Therefore *dermat/ologist* means

_____.

puncture of the abdominal cavity (to drain fluid)

   Abdomino means abdomen;
   -centesis means surgical puncture of a cavity (to drain off fluid).
   Therefore *abdomino/centesis* means

_____.

pertaining to the abdomen and thorax (bony cage of the chest)

25.

The bony cage that forms the chest cavity is called the thorax. What does abdomin/o/thorac/ic mean?

_____

_____.

abdomin/o/
thorac/ic
abdominothoracic
ab dom´ ə nō thō
rā´ sik

26.

A word that means, literally, pertaining to the abdomen and chest cavity is

_____ / ___ / _____ / ____.
abdomen   thorax   pertaining to

thorac/ic
thoracic
thō rā´ sik

27.
Thorac/o forms words about the thorax, or chest cavity. A word that means pertaining to the chest cavity is _____ / _____ .
  thorax   pertaining to

thorac/otomy
thoracotomy
thōr ə kot´ ə mē

28.
Write a word that means incision of the chest cavity: _____ / _____ .

thorac/o centesis
thoracocentesis
thōr´ ə kō sen tē´
  sis

29.
Write a word that means surgical tapping of the chest cavity to remove fluids:
_____ / ___ / _____ .
  thorax   puncture of

thorac/o/plast/y
thoracoplasty
thōr´ ə kō plas´ tē

30.
A word for the surgical repair of the chest cage is _____ / ___ / plast / y .

cyst/o/plast/y
cystoplasty
sis´ tō plas´ tē

31.
Now write a word for surgical repair of a bladder:
_____ / ___ / _____ .

water, fluid, or a
  watery fluid

32.
A hydr/o/cyst is a sac (or bladder) filled with watery fluid. Hydr/o is used in words to mean
_____ .

a collection of
  fluid in the
  head

33.
What does hydr/o/cephal/us mean?
_____
_____ .

hydr/o/cephal/us
hydrocephalus
hī′ drō sə fal′ us

34.
A disease characterized by an enlarged head due to an increased amount of fluid in the skull is called _____/____/_____/ us .
  water   head

hydrocephalus

35.
Unless arrested, accumulated fluid in the head results in deformity of the cranium. The face seems small. The eyes are abnormal. Increased pressure and brain damage may result from _____.

abnormal fear

36.
Hydr/o/phob/ia means having an abnormal fear of water. Phob/ia means _____.

hydr/o/phob/ia
hydrophobia
hī drō fō′ bē ə

37.
An abnormal fear of water is _____/____/_____/ .

hydrophobia

38.
Some parents are abnormally afraid to have their children swim or even ride in a boat. These parents suffer from _____.

hydr/o/therap/y
hydrotherapy
hī′ drō ther′ ə pē

39.
Therap/y means treatment. Treatment by water is _____/____/_____/ .

hydrotherapy

40.
Swirling water baths are a form of _____.

41.
The pelvis is formed by the pelvic bones. To find the measurement of a woman's pelvis during pregnancy, the physician does pelv/i/metr/y. What part of the word refers to measurement of?

metr   _____.

42.
To determine whether a woman has a pelvis large enough to avoid trouble during labor, a physician can measure the pelvic bones. This measurement

pelvimetry   is called _____.
pel vim´ ə trē

43.
a measuring   What do you think a pelvimeter is?
    device used for   _____
    pelvimetry (or   _____.
    equivalent)

44.
When a physician measures the patient's pelvis,
pelvimetry   the doctor is doing _____.
pelvimeter   The instrument used is a _____.

45.
surgical repair of   Crani/o is used in words referring to the crani/um
    the skull or   or skull. Crani/o/plast/y means _____
    cranium   _____.

46.
crani/ectomy   Write a medical term for each of the following:
craniectomy   excision of part of the cranium,
krā nē ek´ tō mē   _____/_____ ;
                    skull   excision of

crani/otomy
craniotomy   incision into the skull,
krā nē ot´ ō mē   _____/_____ ;
                    cranium   incision into

(Continued on next page)

crani/o/meter
craniometer

an instrument to measure the cranium,
_____/ /_____.

47.
The cerebrum (cerebr/o) is where thought occurs.
What is the meaning of crani/o/cerebr/al?

of, or pertaining
   to, the brain and
   skull

_____

_____.

48.
Have you ever been told to use your "gray matter"?
Gray matter controls thinking, feeling, and
movement. The gray matter is the largest part of

brain, or cerebrum

the _____.

cerebr/al
cerebral
ser ē´ brəl

49.
Write a term meaning of, or pertaining to, the gray
matter of the brain: _____.

spin/al
spinal
spī´ nəl

50.
Cerebr/o/spin/al refers to the brain and spinal
cord. What part of the word means pertaining to
the spinal cord? _____.

cerebr/o/spin/al
cerebrospinal
ser ē brō spī´ nəl

51.
A puncture or tap to remove fluid from the space
around the cerebrum and spinal cord is called a
spinal tap or _____/ /_____/ al
puncture.   cerebrum   spinal

cocc

52.
Let's try some different ones. Cocc/i is the plural of
cocc/us. When building words about a whole
family of bacteria, the cocci, use the word root

_____.

(See Appendix B for more information on the
formation of plurals.)

53.

cocc/i
kok' sī

Pneumonia is caused by the pneumococcus. From this you know that the germ responsible for pneumonia belongs to the family _____/____
(plural).

54.

There are three main types of coccus:
cocci growing in pairs are

dipl/o/cocc/i

___dipl___ / o / _____ / ____;
cocci growing in twisted chains are

strept/o/cocc/i

___strept___ / o / _____ / ___;
cocci growing in clusters are

staphyl/o/cocc/i

___staphyl___ / o / _____ / ____.

55.

strept/o/cocc/i
strep' tō kok' sī

If you should see a twisted chain of cocci when examining a slide under a microscope, you would say they were _____/ / _____/ ___.

56.

staphyl/o/cocc/i
staphylococci
staf' i lō kok' sī

Staphyle is the Greek word for bunch of grapes. If you should see a cluster of cocci when using a microscope, you would say they were _____/ / _____.

57.

staphylococci

The bacteria that cause carbuncles grow in clusters like a bunch of grapes. Carbuncles are caused by _____.

58.

producing pus

Py/o is the root used for words involving pus. Genesis (gen/o) is from a Greek word meaning produce or originate. Py/o/gen/ic means _____.

py/o/gen/ic
pyogenic

59.
Staphylococci produce pus; therefore, they are
_____ / ___ / _____ / ic .

pyogenic

60.
Bacteria that form pus are referred to as
_____ .

pyogenic

61.
Boils are purulent (contain pus). This pus is
formed by _____ bacteria.
                    pus-producing

discharge of pus

62.
The suffix -orrhea means flow or discharge.
Py/orrhea means _____
_____ .

py/orrhea
pyorrhea
pī ō rē´ ə

63.
The suffix -orrhea refers to any flow or discharge.
A flow of pus is called _____ / _____ .

pyorrhea

64.
Pyorrhea alveolaris is a disease of the teeth and
gums. The word that tells you pus is being
discharged is _____ .

pyorrhea

65.
When pus flows from the salivary gland, the
disease is called _____ salivaris.

ear

66.
Ot/orrhea means a discharging ear; ot/o is the root
for _____ .

ot/orrhea otorrhea ō tō rē′ ə	**67.** Ot/orrhea is both a symptom and a disease. No matter which is meant, the word to use is _____/_____. ear discharge
otorrhea	**68.** This disease involves discharge, inflammation, and deafness. One of its symptoms is also its name, _____.
inflammation of the middle ear	**69.** Otorrhea may be a sign of ot/itis media. Ot/itis media means _____
ot/algia otalgia	**70.** Otitis usually causes ear pain. The medical term is _____/_____. ear pain
otalgia	**71.** Small children often complain of an earache. Medically this could be called _____.
nose	**72.** Rhinorrhea means discharge from the nose. Rhin/o is used in words about the _____.
rhin/itis rhinitis rī nī′ tis	**73.** Taking what is necessary from rhin/o, form a word that means inflammation of the nose: _____/_____.

rhin/orrhea
rhinorrhea

74.
Drainage from the nose due to a head cold is a symptom called _____ / _____ .

rhinorrhea

75.
Discharge from the sinuses through the nose is a form of _____ .

rhin/o/plast/y
rhinoplasty

76.
Build a word that means surgical repair of the nose: _____ / __ / _____ / ____ .

rhin/otomy
rhinotomy

Form a word that means incision into the nose:
_____ / _____ .

calculus or stone

77.
A rhin/o/lith is a calculus or stone in the nose. Lith/o is the combining form for _____
_____ .

calculi (calculus)
or stones

78.
Lithogenesis means producing or forming
_____ .

lith/otomy
lithotomy
lith ot´ə mē

79.
Taking what is necessary from lith/o, build a word meaning an incision for the removal of a stone:
_____ / _____ .
stone   incision into (for)

gall or bile

80.
Calculi or stones form in many places in the body. A chol/e/lith is a gallstone. Chol/e is the word root for _____ .

81.

chol/e/lith
cholelith

One cause of gallbladder disease is the presence of
a gallstone or _____ / / _____ .
                        gall   stone

82.

cholelith

No matter what its size or shape, irritation and
blockage of the gallbladder can be caused by a
_____ .

83.

gallbladder

Gall is the fluid secreted by the gallbladder.
Chol/e/cyst is a medical name for the
_____ .

84.

chol/e/cyst/itis
cholecystitis
kō′ lē sis tī′ tis

When gallstones result in inflammation of the
gallbladder, this condition is called
_____ / / _____ / _____ .
gall   bladder   inflammation

85.

cholecystitis

Cholecystitis is accompanied by pain and emesis.
Fatty foods aggravate these symptoms and should
be avoided in cases of _____ .

86.

cholecystitis

Butter, cream, and whole milk contain fat and
should be avoided by patients with
_____ .

chol/e/cyst/otomy
cholecystotomy
kō lē sis tot´ e mē
or
chol/e/lith/otomy
cholelithotomy
kō´ lē lith ot´ ə mē

87.
When a cholelith causes cholecystitis, one of two surgical procedures may solve the problem. One is an incision into the gallbladder to remove stones, called a _____ / / _____ / _____ .

chol/e/cyst/ectomy
cholecystectomy
kō´ lē sis tek´ tō
mē

88.
More often, the presence of a gallstone calls for excision of the gallbladder, called
_____ / / _____ / _____ .

89.
It's time to review. From List B select the best meaning for each term in List A. Write your choice in the space provided.

	List A	List B
pelvis	pelv/i _____	measure
stone, calculus	lith/o_____	skull
gall, bile	chol/e_____	pus
pus	py/o _____	pelvis
skull	crani/o _____	cerebrum
cerebrum	cerebr/o _____	gall, bile
measure	metr/o _____	stone, calculus
nose	rhin/o_____	chainlike
ear	ot/o _____	double
chainlike	strept/o_____	chest
grapelike	staphyl/o _____	bladder
double	dipl/o _____	nose
chest	thorac/o _____	ear
bladder, sac	cyst/o _____	grapelike

90.
Complete the following:

away from   The prefix ab- means _____ the midline.
toward   The prefix ad- means _____ the midline.
fluid, water   The prefix hydro- means_____.

91.
Select the best meaning for each of the following word parts.

treatment   therapy _____   surgical puncture
calculus, stone   lith _____   abnormal fear
discharge, flow   orrhea _____   calculus, stone
surgical puncture   centesis_____   treatment
abnormal fear   phobia_____   discharge, flow

92.
Suffixes create adjectives when used with a word root. The new word means of, or pertaining to (the word root). Write the meaning of each term.

SUFFIXES	EXAMPLE	MEANING
-al	duoden/al	_____
-ic	gastr/ic	_____
-ar	lumb/ar	_____
-ac	cardi/ac	_____

93.

Here are more than 35 new medical terms you formed in Unit 3. Read them one at a time and pronounce each aloud.

aberrant (ab er´ ant)

abdominal (ab dom´ i nəl)

abdominocentesis
    (ab dom´ i nō sen tē´ sis)

abduction (ab duk´ shun)

adduction (ad duk´ shun)

cardiocentesis (kär´ dē ō sen tē´ sis)

cerebral (ser ē´ brəl)

cerebrospinal (ser ē brō spī´ nəl)

cholecystectomy
    (kō´ lē sis tek´ tō mē)

cholecystitis (kō´ lē sis tī´ tis)

cholelithotomy (kō´ lē lith ot´ ə mē)

craniectomy (krā nē ek´ tō mē)

cranioplasty (krā´ nē ō plas´ tē)

craniotomy (krā nē ot´ ō mē)

cranium (krā´ nē um)

cystitis (sis tī´ tis)

cystocele (sis´ to sēl)

cystotomy (sis tot´ ə mē)

diplococci (dip´ lō kok´ sī)

hydrocephalus (hī´ drō sə fal´ us)

hydrotherapy (hī´ drō ther´ ə pē)

lithotomy (lith ot´ ō mē)

otalgia (ō tal´ jē a)

otitis (ō tī´ tis)

otorrhea (ō tō rē´ ə)

pelvic (pel´ vik)

pelvimetry (pel vim´ ə trē)

pyogenic (pī ō jen´ ik)

pyorrhea (pī ō rē´ ə)

rhinitis (rī nī´ tis)

rhinoplasty (rī´ nō plas tē)

rhinorrhea (rī nōr rē´ ə)

staphylococci (staf´ i lō kok´ sī)

thoracic (thō rā´ sik)

thoracocentesis
    (thōr´ ə kō sen tē´ sis)

thoracoplasty (thōr´ ə kō plas´ tē)

thoracotomy (thōr ə kot´ ə mē)

Take the Unit 3 Self-Test before going on.

Unit 3 Self-Test

PART 1

From the list on the right, select the correct meaning for each of the following terms. Write the letter in the space provided.

____ 1. Thoracocentesis	a. Pertaining to the cerebrum and spinal cord
____ 2. Cholelithotomy	b. Relating to the pelvis
____ 3. Otorrhea	c. Wandering or out of the normal place
____ 4. Cystotomy	d. Tapping or puncturing the chest cavity
____ 5. Abdominalgia	e. Movement toward the midline
____ 6. Cranium	f. Abnormal fear of water
____ 7. Cerebrospinal	g. Running or draining from the ear
____ 8. Hydrophobia	h. Incision into the bladder
____ 9. Adduction	i. Producing pus
____ 10. Streptococci	j. The bony vault surrounding the brain
____ 11. Pyogenic	k. Incision for the purpose of removing a gallstone
____ 12. Aberrant	l. Commonly referred to as a "bellyache"
____ 13. Pelvic	m. Cocci bacteria that grow in chains
____ 14. Cholecystotomy	n. Surgical repair of the nose
____ 15. Rhinoplasty	o. Incision into the gallbladder

PART 2

Complete each of the medical terms on the right with the appropriate word root:

1. Herniation of a bladder   _____ cele
2. Tapping or puncturing of the
   heart chamber   _____ centesis

3. Surgical repair of the bony vault
   that encloses the brain   _____ plasty
4. Earache   _____ algia
5. Gallstone   _____ lith
6. Inflammation of the nose   _____ itis
7. Measurement of the pelvis   _____ metry
8. Relating to the thorax   _____ ic
9. Collection of fluid in the head   Hydro _____
10. Incision into the cranium   _____ otomy
11. Relating to the formation
    of pus   _____ genic
12. Surgical repair of the
    chest cage   _____ plasty
13. Instrument for measuring
    the pelvis   _____ meter
14. Relating to the abdomen   _____ al
15. Surgical removal of the
    gallbladder   Chole_____

ANSWERS

Part 1

1. d	9. e
2. k	10. m
3. g	11. i
4. h	12. c
5. l	13. b
6. j	14. o
7. a	15. n
8. f	

Part 2

1. Cystocele	9. Hydrocephalus
2. Cardiocentesis	10. Craniotomy
3. Cranioplasty	11. Pyogenic
4. Otalgia	12. Thoracoplasty
5. Cholelith	13. Pelvimeter
6. Rhinitis	14. Abdominal
7. Pelvimetry	15. Cholecystectomy
8. Thoracic	

Unit 4

In Unit 4 you will make at least 50 new words by using some of the word roots, prefixes, and suffixes you have covered in earlier units. You will also use the following:

angi/o (*vessel*)
arter/i/o (*artery*)
blast/o (*embryo*)
colp/o (*vagina*)
crypt/o (*hidden*)
fibr/o (*fiber*)
hem/o, hemat/o (*blood*)
hyster/o (*uterus*)
kinesi/o (*motion*)
lys/o (*destruction*)
men/o (*menses*)
my/o (*muscle*)
nephr/o (*kidney*)

neur/o (*nerve*)
o/o (*egg, ovum*)
oophor/o (*ovary*)
orchid/o (*testes*)
peps/o, peps/ia (*digestion*)
pne/o (*air, breathe*)
pyel/o (*pelvis of the kidney*)
salping/o (*fallopian tube*)
scler/o (*tough, hard*)
spermat/o (*sperm*)
ureter/o (*ureter*)
urethr/o (*urethra*)
ur/o (*urine*)

a-, an- (*without*)
brady- (*slow*)
dys- (*pain*)
tachy- (*fast*)

-blast (*embryonic*)
-ia (*noun ending*)
-orrhagia (*hemorrhage*)
-orrhaphy (*suture*)
-pexy (*fixation*)
-ptosis (*drooping*)
-spasm (*twitching*)
-sperm (*sperm*)

1.
Brad/y is used in words to mean slow.

slow   Brad/y/cardi/a means _____ heart action.

brad/y/cardi/a
bradycardia
brad ē kär´ dē ə

2.
Abnormally slow heart action is
_____ / ____ / _____ / ____ .

3.
Kinesi/o is used in words to mean movement or
motion. Brad/y/kinesi/a means

slowness of
  movement
_____

_____ .

4.
pain on movement   Kinesi/algia means _____
  or movement
  pain
_____

_____ .

5.
kinesi/algia   When moving any sore or injured part of the body,
kinesialgia   pain occurs. Moving a broken arm causes
kin ē´ sē al´ jē ə
_____ / _____ .

6.
                After a first ride on horseback, almost any
kinesialgia   movement causes _____ .

7.
kinesi/o/logy   The suffix -ology means study of. (Remember
kinesiology   o/logist?) The study of muscular movements is
kin ē´ sē ol´ ə jē
_____ / ____ / _____ .

8.
                Kinesi/o/logy is the study of movement. The study
                of muscular movement during exercise is known as
kinesiology   the scientific field of _____ .

9.

kinesiology

The whole science of how the body moves is embraced in the field of _____.

10.

abnormally slow
  movement

Brad/y/kinesi/a means _____

_____.

11.

abnormally fast
  or rapid heart
  action

Tach/y is used in words to show the opposite of slow. Thus tach/y/card/ia means _____

_____

_____.

tach/y/cardi/a
tachycardia
tak ə kär´ dē ə

12.

Write the medical term for an abnormally fast heartbeat: _____ / / _____ / __.

13.

breathe or
  breathing

Pne/o comes from the Greek word *pneia* (breathe). Pne/o any place in a word means

_____.

14.

will
brad ip nē´ ə

silent

When pne/o begins a word, the "p" is silent. When pne/o occurs later in a word, the "p" is pronounced; for example, when you pronounce brad/y/pne/a, you _____ pronounce the

                       (will/will not)

"p." In the term pneu/mon/ia, the "p" is

_____.

  (pronounced/silent)

slow
  breathing

15.
Brad/y/pne/a means _____
_____.

tach/y/pne/a
tachypnea
tak ip nē´ ə

A word for rapid breathing is
_____.

tachypnea

16.
The rate of respiration (breathing) is controlled by
the amount of carbon dioxide in the blood.
Increased carbon dioxide speeds up breathing and
causes _____.

tachypnea

17.
Muscle exercise increases the amount of carbon
dioxide in the blood. This speeds respiration and
produces _____.

without
  breathing

18.
The prefix *a*- literally means without. Thus apnea
means _____
_____.

a/pne/a
apnea
ap´ nē ə

19.
A/pnea really means temporary cessation of
breathing. If the failure to breathe were not
temporary, death would result. Temporary
cessation of breathing is referred to as
__ / _____ / __ .

apnea

20.
If the level of carbon dioxide in the blood falls very
low, temporary cessation of breathing results. This
is called _____.

bradypnea

21.
If breathing is merely very slow, it is called
_____.

tachypnea
a-

22.
When breathing is abnormally fast, it is called
_____. The prefix meaning without
is _____.

dys/pne/a
dyspnea
disp´ nē ə

23.
The prefix dys- means painful, bad, or difficult.
Dys/troph/y literally means bad development.
Write a word for difficult breathing:
_____ / _____ / ___.

dys-

24.
Dys/men/orrhea means painful menstruation. The
prefix for painful, bad, or difficult is _____.

poor or painful
digestion

25.
Pepsis (peps/o) is the Greek word for digestion.
Dys/peps/ia means _____
_____.

dys/peps/ia
dyspepsia
dis pep´ sē ə

26.
Eating under tension may cause painful or poor
digestion. This is called _____ / _____ / ___.

dyspepsia

27.
Contemplating the troubles of the world while
eating is a good cause for _____.

28.
Here's a quick review of what you just covered.
From List B select the best meaning for each term
in List A. Write your choice in the space provided.

	List A		List B
menses	men/o _____		digestion
digestion	peps/o _____		movement
breathe, breathing	pne/o _____		menses
movement	kinesi/o _____		breathe, breathing

29.
Try these.

	List A		List B
painful	dys- _____		very slow
very slow	brady- _____		painful
abnormally fast	tachy- _____		without, absence of
without, absence of	a- _____		abnormally fast

30.
Build a word for each of the following definitions
using a prefix you just learned.

a/pnea	absence of breath _____ / _____
tachy/cardia	fast heartbeat _____ / _____
brady/kinesia	slow movement _____ / _____
dys/pepsia	painful digestion _____ / _____

Refer to the table below to work through frames 31 to 41.

SOME COMBINING FORMS

angi/o	vessel, blood & lymphatic
arteri/o	artery
fibr/o	fibrous, fiber
hem/o, hemat/o	blood
malac/o	soft, softened
lip/o	fat
my/o	muscle
neur/o	nerve or neuron
scler/o	hard

SOME SUFFIXES

-lysis	declining, dissolution
-spasm	twitch, twitching
-blast	germ or embryonic
-osis	condition of
-oma	tumor
-ia, -y	these endings make the term a noun

---

neur/o/blast
neuroblast
nyo͞o´ ro blast

31.
An embryonic (germ) cell from which a muscle develops is a my/o/blast. A germ cell from which a nerve cell develops is a

_____/ / _____.

angi/o/blast
angioblast
an´ jē ō blast

32.
A germ cell from which vessels develop is an

_____/ / _____.

my/o/spasm
myospasm
mī´ ō spa zm

33.
A spasm of a nerve is a neur/o/spasm.
A spasm of a muscle is a
_____/___/_____ .

angi/o/spasm
angiospasm
an´ jē ō spa´ zm

A spasm of a vessel is an
_____/___/_____ .

angi/o/scler/osis
angiosclerosis
an´ jē ō sklə rō´ sis

34.
A (condition of) hardening of nerve tissue is
neur/o/scler/osis. A hardening of a vessel is
_____/___/_____/_____ .

my/o/scler/osis
myosclerosis
mī´ ō sklə rō´ sis

A hardening of muscle tissue is
_____/___/_____/_____ .

neur/o/fibr/oma
neurofibroma
nyōō´ rō´ fī brō´ mä

35.
A tumor containing muscle and fibrous connective
tissue is a my/o/fibr/oma. A tumor containing
fibrous connective tissue and nerve tissue is a
_____/___/_____/___ .

angi/o/fibr/oma
angiofibroma
an´ jē ō fī brō´ mä

A vessel tumor containing fibrous connective
tissue is a(n) _____/___/_____/___ .

neur/o/lys/is
neurolysis
nyōō rol´ ə sis

36.
The destruction of muscle tissue is my/o/lys/is.
The destruction of nerve tissue is
_____/___/_____/___ .

angi/o/lys/is
angiolysis
an jē ol´ i sis

The destruction or breaking down of vessels is
_____/___/_____/___ .

arteri/o/scler/osis
arteriosclerosis
ar ter´ ē ō skler ō´
    sis

37.
Refer to the table only when you must. Arteri/o is
used in words about the arteries. A word meaning
hardening of the arteries is
_____/___/_____/_____.

arteri/o/skler/osis
arteriosclerosis

arteri/o/malac/ia
arteriomalacia
ar ter´ ē ō mä lā´
    zha

38.
Build a word meaning a hardened condition of the
arteries: _____/___/_____/_____.

A softened artery is called
_____/___/_____/_____.

arteri/o/spasm
arteriospasm
ar ter´ ē ō spa´ zm

lip/o/lys/is
lipolysis
lip ol´ i sis

39.
Build a word meaning arterial spasm:
_____/___/_____.

Dissolution (breakdown) of fat is called
_____/___/_____/____.

hem/angi/itis
hemangiitis
hē man´ jē ī tis

hem/o/lysis
hemolysis
hē mol´ ə sis

40.
Hem/o refers to blood. A tumor of a blood vessel is
a hem/angi/oma . (Note dropped o.) An
inflammation of a blood vessel is
_____/_____/_____.

Breaking down of blood tissue (cells) is
_____/___/_____.

hemat/o/logy
hematology
hē mə tol´ ə jē

hemat/o/logist
hematologist
hē mə tol´ ə jist

41.
Hemat/o also refers to blood. The study of blood
is _____/___/_____.

One who specializes in the science of blood is a
_____/___/_____.

42.

Let´s go over the new material again briefly. Match the best definition in List B with the word root in List A. Write your selection in the space provided.

	List A	List B
artery	arteri/o _____	fat
fibrous connective tissue	fibr/o_____	muscle
blood	hem/o, hemat/o _____	artery
fat	lip/o _____	blood and lymph vessel
soften	malac/o _____	soften
muscle	my/o _____	harden
nerve	neur/o _____	fibrous connective tissue
harden	scler/o _____	blood
blood and lymph vessel	angi/o _____	nerve

Now match the best definition in List B with the suffix in List A. Write the term.

	List A	List B
destruction of	-lysis _____	tumor
twitching	-spasm _____	science, or study of
tumor	-oma _____	condition of
inflammation of	-itis _____	twitching
germ cell (immature)	-blast _____	inflammation of
condition of	-osis _____	destruction of
science, or study of	-ology _____	germ cell (immature)

43.

Build a word for each of the following definitions.

arterio/scler/osis	a condition of hardening of the arteries	_____ / _____ / _____
hemat/oma	blood tumor	_____ / _____
angio/spasm	blood vessel spasm	_____ / _____
myo/fibr/oma	fibrous muscle tumor	_____ / _____ / _____
neuro/blast	nerve tissue germ cell	_____ / _____
lipo/lysis	breakdown of fat tissue	_____ / _____

The Male Genital Organs

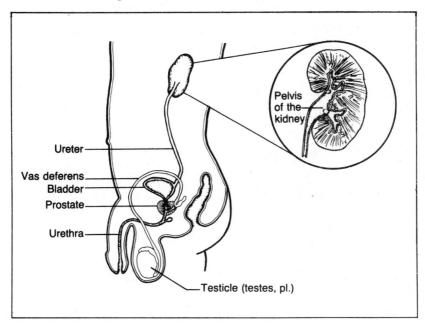

Ureter

Vas deferens
Bladder
Prostate

Urethra

Pelvis
of the
kidney

Testicle (testes, pl.)

Refer to the illustration as you work through frames 44 to 55.

44.
The testes are organs that manufacture the male germ cells; that is, spermatozoa are formed in the

testes (pl.)   _____.

45.
Orchid/algia means pain in a testicle or testis.
excision of a   Orchid/ectomy means _____
testicle, testis   _____.

orchid/itis
orchiditis
or ki dī´ tis

46.
Build a word meaning inflammation of a testicle,
_____ / _____ ;

orchid/otomy
orchidotomy
or kid ot´ ō mē

incision into a testis,
_____ / _____ .

47.
A crypt/ic remark is one with a hidden meaning. A
crypt/ic belief is obscure. The word root for hidden

crypt
kript´

or obscure is _____ .

crypt/orchid/ism
cryptorchidism
kript ôr´ kid ism

48.
Near the time of birth the testes of the fetus
normally descend from the abdominal cavity into
the scrotum. Sometimes this fails to happen, and
the testes are not evident at birth. This condition of
undescended testes is called
_____ / _____ / ism .
        hidden   testicle

cryptorchidism

49.
When a testis is hidden in the abdominal cavity,
the condition is called _____ .

orchid/o/(pexy)

50.
An operation to repair the condition is called
orchid/o/pexy. Circle the part of the term that
means to fix the testes in their proper place.

formation of
  spermatozoa,
  sperm, or male
  germ cells

51.
Sperma is the Greek word meaning seed.
Spermat/o is used in words about spermat/o/zoa
or male germ cells (sperm). Spermat/o/genesis
means _____
_____ .

spermat/o/lysis
spermatolysis
sperm´ ə tol´ i sis

52.
Give a word meaning the destruction of
spermatozoa, _____ / / _____ ;

spermat/o/blast
spermatoblast
sper mat´ ō blast

an embryonic male cell,
_____ / / _____ ;

spermat/oid
spermatoid
sper´ mä toid

resembling sperm,
_____ / _____ .

53.
Summarize what you learned:

muscle   my/o   means _____ ,
vessel   angi/o   means _____ ,
nerve   neur/o   means _____ .

54.
Again.

twitching   spasm   means _____ ,
germ or embryonic   blast/o   means _____ ,
hard   scler/o   means _____ ,
fibrous   fibr/o   means _____ ,
destruction of   lysis   means _____ .

55.
And these.

spermatozoa (sperm) spermat/o means _____ ,
blood   hemat/o   means _____ ,
blood   hem/o   means _____ ,
formation of   genesis   means _____ .

Correct any definitions you may have missed; then
cover the word roots, read the definitions you have
written, and write the appropriate word root in the
right-hand margin.

The Female Genital Organs

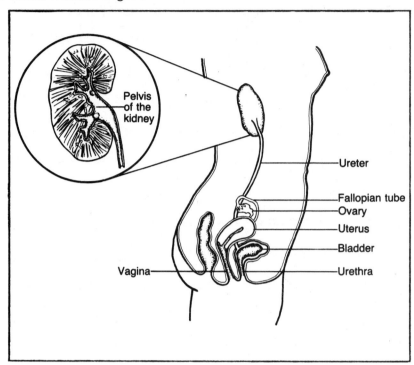

Refer to the illustration as you work through frames 56 to 77.

56.
The Greek word for egg is *oon*. In scientific words, o/o (pronounce both o's) means egg or ovum. An o/o/blast is _____ _____ _____.

an embryonic egg cell (a cell that will become an ovum)

57.
An ovum is discharged from the ovary. The root used in words referring to the ovary is oophor/o. What does oophor/ectomy mean?

excision, or surgical removal of the ovary
_____ _____.

58.

oophor/itis
oophoritis
ōō fôr ī′ tis

Using what you need from oophor/o, build a word that means inflammation of an ovary:
_____/_____.

59.

oophor/ectomy
oophorectomy
ōō fôr ek′ tō mē

Build a term for each of the following:
excision of an ovary,
_____/_____;

oophor/oma
oophoroma
ōō fôr ō′ ma

tumor of an ovary (ovarian tumor),
_____/_____.

60.

fixation (of)

Oophoropexy means fixation of a displaced ovary. Pex/o is a root meaning _____.

61.

oophor/o/pex/y
oophoropexy
ōō′ fôr ō pek′ sē

When an ovary is displaced, a surgical procedure to fix it back in its normal place is called
_____/ _____/_____.

62.

oophoropexy

The surgical procedure for a prolapsed (dropped or sagging) ovary is called an
_____.

63.

fallopian tube(s)

Salping/o is used to build words that refer to the fallopian tube(s). A salpingoscope is an instrument used to examine the
_____.

64.

salping/itis
salpingitis
sal pin jī´ tis

Using what you need of salping/o, build a word meaning inflammation of a fallopian tube,

_____ / _____ ;

salping/ectomy
salpingectomy
sal pin jek´ tō mē

excision of a fallopian tube,

_____ / _____ ;

salping/ostomy
salpingostomy
sal pin gos´ tō mē

a permanent opening into a fallopian tube,

_____ / _____ .

65.

In words built from laryng/o, pharyng/o, and salping/o, the "g" is pronounced as a hard "g" when followed by an "o" or an "a." The "g" in good is a hard "g"; for example, in laryngalgia and salpingocele, the "g" of the word root is pronounced hard as in _____ .

game and good
(pronounce
them)

(game/good) or (germ/giant)

66.

In laryngostomy, pharyngotomy, and salpingopexy, the "g" is followed by an "o" and is a _____ sound.

hard (pronounce
them)

(hard/soft)

67.

"o" and "a"

A hard "g" precedes the vowels _____ and _____ .

68.

In words built from laryng/o, pharyng/o, and salping/o, the "g" is soft when followed by an "e" or an "i"; for example, in laryngectomy and salpingitis, the "g" is soft as in _____ .

germ and giant
(pronounce
them)

(game/good) or (germ/giant)

69.
In salpingian, laryngitis, and pharyngectomy,
the "g" is given a _____ sound because it
                    (soft/hard)
precedes the vowels _____ and _____.

soft (pronounce
   them)
"e" and "i"

laryngⒹctomy
pharyngalgia
pharyngⒺtis
salpingo-
   oophorectomy

70.
Circle the vowels in each of the following words
which mean that the "g" is given the soft "j" sound:
laryngectomy   pharyngitis
pharyngalgia   salpingo-oophorectomy

salping/o-/oophor/
   itis
salpingo-oophoritis
sal´ pin gō ōō fôr
   ī´ tis

71.
In compound medical words, if two like vowels
occur between word roots, they are separated by a
hyphen. Use salpingo-oophorectomy as a model
and build a word that means inflammation of the
fallopian tube and ovary:
_____ / / _____ / ____.

two like vowels
   join word roots

72.
In compound words, a hyphen (-) is used when
_____
_____
_____.

inflammation of
   the vagina

73.
Colp/o is used in words about the vagina. Colpitis
means
_____.

74.
A colp/o/spasm is a

vaginal spasm   _____.

colp/otomy
colpotomy   Incision into the vagina is a
kôl pot´ ō mē   _____/_____.

75.
colp/o/plasty   Build a word meaning surgical repair of the vagina,
    (you pronounce)   _____/_____/_____/___;

colp/o/scope
colposcope   instrument for examining the vagina,
kôl´ pō skōp   _____/_____/_____.

76.
Hyster/o is used to build words about the uterus.
A hyster/ectomy is an excision of the

uterus   _____.

77.
Write words for the following:
an incision into the uterus,
hysterotomy   _____;

a spasm of the uterus,
hysterospasm   _____;

surgical fixation of the uterus,
hysteropexy   _____.

78.
Some terms are composed of many word roots plus
a prefix and a suffix. These terms usually list the
parts of the body in a special order.

For example, when you swallow food it passes
from the esophagus to the stomach to the
duodenum. So when a physician takes a look
inside the digestive system with an endoscope the
procedure is called
        esophago / gastro / duoden / oscopy

Follow the same order and build a word that
means inflammation of the stomach and
gastroduodenitis   duodenum, _____.

79.
Examination of the female genital system begins at
the vulva, then the vagina, to the uterus, fallopian
tubes, and ovaries.

Follow the same order and build a word that
means an operation to remove uterus, fallopian
hystero/salpingo/   tubes, and ovaries:
oophor/ectomy
_____

Of course , prefixes still come in front of the word.

80.

Stop here and summarize what you've just covered. Match the best definition in List B with the word root in List A. Write your selection in the space provided.

	List A	List B
ovary	oophor/o _____	fallopian tubes
male germ cells	spermat/o _____	vagina
uterus	hyster/o _____	male germ cells
fallopian tubes	salping/o _____	egg, ovum
testicle	orchid/o _____	hidden
vagina	colp/o _____	testicle
egg, ovum	o/o _____	ovary
hidden	crypt _____	uterus
surgical fixation	-pexy _____	resembling
produce, originate	-genesis _____	twitching
resembling	-oid _____	suturing to repair
twitching	-spasm _____	produce, originate
embryo, germ cell	-blast _____ ____	embryo, germ cell
suturing to repair	-orrhaphy _____	surgical fixation

81.

Build a word for each of the following:

suturing (to repair) the vagina,

colp/orrhaphy   _____ / _____;

spasm of the uterus,

hyster/o/spasm   _____ / _____;

fixation of the testes,

orchido/pexy   _____ / _____;

inflammation of ovary and fallopian tube,

salpingo/oophor/   _____ / _____ / _____;
itis

formation of spermatozoa,

spermato/genesis   _____ / _____;

embryonic male germ cell,

spermato/blast   _____ / _____.

82.

Now let´s have some fun. Read each term and its meaning. Then study the accompanying illustrations.

The protrusion of an organ or part of an organ through the wall of the cavity that normally contains it is a rupture, or a *hernia*.

A sinking down or sagging of an organ or part (from its normal position) is *ptosis*.

An irregularity, that is, when an organ or structure is abnormal or contrary to the general rule, is a condition called an *anomaly*.

Localized abnormal dilation of a blood vessel, or ballooning out of the vessel at a weak point, is an *aneurysm*.

Write the correct term below each illustration:

A. anomaly
B. aneurysm
C. hernia
D. ptosis

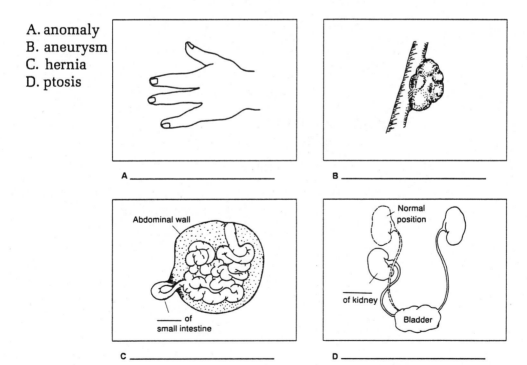

A _____

B _____

C _____

D _____

83.

sinking down,
prolapse, or
sagging

Hyster/o/ptosis means prolapse (sagging) or sinking down of the uterus. Ptosis (pronounced tō´ sis) is a word that means _____.

84.

hyster/o/ptosis
hysteroptosis
his´ ter op´ tō sis

When prolapse occurs, the uterus may be surgically fixed in its normal place. A hysteropexy would be done to correct or repair the condition known as _____ / ___ / _____.

85.

From the terms provided, select one that best fits each definition.

anomaly   hernia   aneurysm   ptosis

Protrusion of an organ or part through the wall of the cavity in which it is normally enclosed.

hernia

_____

The sagging of an organ or part from its normal position.

ptosis

_____

The abnormal ballooning out of a blood vessel at a weak point.

aneurysm

_____

Irregularity in structure of an organ or part; the structure is contrary to the general rule.

anomaly

_____

86.
Fill in the missing words to complete each of the following definitions.

Ptosis is the sagging of an organ or part from its

normal

_____ position.

Hernia is the protrusion of an organ or part through

wall

the _____ of a cavity that
normally contains it.

Anomaly is an irregularity. It is an organ or
structure that is contrary to the general

rule

_____.

Aneurysm is the abnormal ballooning out of a

vessel

_____ at a weak point.

87.
Complete each of the following descriptions by
writing the form of the term that fits best.

An irregular organ or structure that is contrary to

anomalous
 (adjective)

the general rule is said to be

_____.

When an organ or part protrudes through the wall
of the cavity that normally contains it, we say it has

herniated (verb)

_____.

When a weak spot in the wall of the aorta (artery)
balloons out, we call it an aortic

aneurysm (noun)

_____.

Nephr/o is used in words that refer to the kidney.
If a kidney sags from its normal position, the
condition is referred to as nephr/o/

nephroptosis

_____.

88.
Label each illustration below.

A. hernia
B. anomaly
C. ptosis
D. aneurysm

Abdominal wall

_____ of
small intestine

A _____

B _____

Normal
position

_____
of kidney

Bladder

C _____

D _____

We suggest something like these:

aneurysm: an abnormal ballooning out of a vessel at a weak point.

anomaly: an organ or structure that is contrary to the rule.

hernia: protrusion of an organ or part through the wall that normally contains it.

ptosis: sagging of an organ or part from its normal location.

In your own words, write a brief definition for each of the following terms.

aneurysm: _____
_____
_____ .

anomaly: _____
_____
_____ .

hernia: _____
_____
_____ .

ptosis: _____
_____
_____ .

Use the table below to work through frames 90 to 106.

WORD	WORD ROOT	NEW SUFFIX TO USE WHEN NEEDED*
urine kidney	ur/o nephr/o	-orrhaphy (*suturing or stitching*)
renal pelvis ureter	pyel/o ureter/o	-orrhagia (*hemorrhage or "bursting forth" of blood*)
bladder urethra	cyst/o urethr/o	*Note: These two involve combining forms starting with orrh that can be used as suffixes.

89.
Let's go on to a new, but related area. Here is a brief summary of the functions of each part of the urinary tract.

kidney: forms urine;
renal pelvis: collects urine in the kidney;
ureter: carries urine to the bladder;
bladder: stores urine until voiding;
urethra: discharges urine from the body.

90.
The urinary system is responsible for making urine from waste materials in the blood and carrying urine from the body. What is the word root for urine? _____. What is the combining form? _____.

ur
ur/o

renal pelvis

91.
Pyel/o refers to the _____.

pyel/itis
pyelitis
pī ə lī´ tis

92.
Taking what you need from the combining form for renal pelvis, form words meaning inflammation of the renal pelvis, _____/_____;

pyel/o/plast/y
pyeloplasty
pī´ lō plas tē

surgical repair of the renal pelvis,
_____/ / _____/__.

abnormal
   condition of the
   renal pelvis and
   kidney

93.
Pyel/o/nephr/osis means _____
_____
_____.

pyel/o/nephr/itis
pyelonephritis
pī´ lō nef rī´ tis

Form a word that means inflammation of the renal pelvis and kidney:
_____/ / _____/_____.

stone or calculus in
   the ureter

94.
Ureter/o/lith means _____
_____.

ureter/o/lith/o/
   tomy
ureterolithotomy

Form a word that means incision into the ureter (for removal of a stone):
_____/ / _____/ / _____.

surgical repair of
   the ureter and
   renal pelvis

95.
Ureter/o/pyel/o/plast/y means _____
_____
_____.

ureter/o/pyel/itis
ureteropyelitis
yōō rē´ ter ō pī ə lī´
   tis

96.
Form a word meaning inflammation of the ureter and renal pelvis,
_____/ / _____/_____;

ureter/o/cyst/
    ostomy
ureterocystostomy
yōō rē′ ter ō sis tos′
    tō mē
	making a permanent opening between the ureter
	and bladder,
	_____/__/_____/_____.

suturing or
    stitching (for
    the purpose of
    repair, especially
    after trauma)
	97.
	Ureter/orrhaphy introduces a new word part:
	Orrhaphy is not really a suffix, but again (for
	simplification) it can be used as one. Orrhaphy
	means _____.

ureter/orrhaphy ureterorrhaphy yer rē ter ôr′ ə fē	**98.** Form a word meaning suturing of the ureter, _____/_____;
nephr/orrhaphy nephrorrhaphy nef rôr′ ə fē	suturing of a kidney, _____/_____;
cyst/orrhaphy cystorrhaphy sis tôr′ ə fē	suturing the bladder, _____/_____;
neur/orrhaphy neurorrhaphy nyōō rôr′ ə fē	suturing of a nerve, _____/_____.

carries urine from
    the body or
    removes urine
    from the bladder
	99.
	The urethra is the organ that _____
	_____
	_____.

urethr/o	The word root for urethra is _____/____.
suturing of the urethra	**100.** Urethr/orrhaphy means _____ _____.

urethr/otomy
urethrotomy
yer ə throt´ ə mē

101.
Form a word that means incision into the urethra,
_____/_____ ;

urethr/o/spasm
urethrospasm
yer rē´ thrō spasm

spasm of the urethra,
_____/___/_____ .

102.
Another complex word part is orrhagia, which can
be used as a suffix when it follows a word root and
ends a word; orrhagia means

hemorrhage or
  bursting forth of
  blood

_____

_____

_____ .

cyst/orrhagia
cystorrhagia
sis tō rä´ jē ə

103.
Build a word that means hemorrhage of the
bladder, _____/_____ ;

ureter/orrhagia
ureterorrhagia
yer rē´ ter ō rä´ jē ə

hemorrhage of the ureter,
_____/_____ .

104.
Di/a is the combining form meaning pass through
or secrete freely.
Define:

How does the
  dictionary define
  these terms?

diuresis _____ .
diuretic _____ .
dialysis _____ .

105.

Let's have a brief review. Select the correct word root from List B. Write your selection in the space provided in List A.

	List A	List B
cyst/o -	stores urine until voiding _____	nephr/o-
aneurysm	ballooning-out vessel _____	pyel/o-
ureter/o-	carries urine to bladder _____	urethr/o-
anomaly	contrary to the rule, irregular _____	ur/o-
pyel/o-	collects urine in the kidney _____	ureter/o-
urethr/o-	discharges urine from body _____	cyst/o-
neur/o-	nerve _____	aneurysm
hernia	protrusion through cavity wall _____	anomaly
ur/o-	urine _____	hernia
nephr/o-	forms urine _____	neur/o-
-plasty	surgical repair (make new) _____	-lith
-ptosis	drooping _____	-plasty
-pexy	fixing in place _____	-ptosis
-lith	stone, calculus _____	-orrhaphy
-orrhaphy	suturing to repair _____	-orrhagia
-ostomy	permanent opening _____	-ostomy
-orrhagia	hemorrhage _____	-spasm
-spasm	twitching, muscle cramp _____	-pexy

106.

Build a word for each of the following definitions.

diseased condition of kidney and renal pelvis

pyelo/nephr/osis   _____/_____/_____

incision to remove calculus from ureter

uretero/lith/otomy   _____/_____/_____

sagging of the kidney

nephro/ptosis   _____/_____

the study of urine and the urinary system

ur/ology   _____/_____

surgical reconnection of the ureter

ureter/orrhaphy   _____/_____

106. *(Continued)*

repair (make new) the kidney

nephro/plasty

_____/_____

hemorrhage from the urinary bladder

cyst/orrhagia

_____/_____

surgical fixing of the kidney in its place

nephro/pexy

_____/_____

107.
Following are 50 of the medical terms you formed in Unit 4. Pronounce each one aloud before going on to Unit 5.

aneurysm (an´yōo rizm)
angioblast (an´jē ō blast)
angiosclerosis (an´jē ō sklə rō´ sis)
anomaly (an om´ə lē)
apnea (ap´ nē ə)
arteriosclerosis
   (ar ter´ ē ō skler ō´ sis)
arteriospasm (ar ter´ ē ō spa´zm)
bradycardia (brad ē kär´ dē ə)
bradypnea (brad ip nē´ ə)
colporrhaphy (kôl pōr´ə fē)
colposcopy (kôl pōs´ kō pē)
cryptorchidism (krip´ ôr kid ism)
cystorrhagia (sis tō rä jē ə)
dysmenorrhea (dis´ men ōr rē´ ə)
dyspepsia (dis pep´sē ə)
dyspnea (disp´ nē ə)
hemangiitis (hē man jē ī´tis)
hematologist (hē mə tol´ ō jist)
hemolysis (hē mol´ ə sis)
hernia (her´ nē ə)
hysteropexy (his´ter ō peks´ ē)
hysterospasm (his´ter ō spa zm)
hysterotomy (his ter ot´ ō mē)
kinesialgia (kin ē´ sē al´ jē ə)
kinesiology (kin ē´ sē ol´ ə jē)
myosclerosis (mī ō skler ō´ sis)

myospasm (mī´ ō spa zm)
nephritis (nef rī´tis)
nephrolith (nef´rō lith)
nephromegaly (nef´rō meg ə lē)
nephroptosis (nef rop tō´ sis)
neurofibroma (nyōo´ rō fī brō´ mä)
neurolysis (nyōo rol´ ə sis)
o-oblast (ō´ō blast)
oophoropexy (ōo´ fôr ō pek´ sē)
orchidotomy (or kid ot´ ō mē)
pyelitis (pī ə lī´ tis)
pyeloplasty (pī ə´ lō plas tē)
salpingectomy (sal pin jek´ tō mē)
salpingo-oophorectomy
   (sal pin´ gō ōo fôr ek´ tō mē)
salpingoscopy (sal pin gos´ kō pē)
spermatoblast (sper mat´ ō blast)
spermatoid (sper´ ma toid)
tachycardia (tak ə kär´ dē ə)
tachypnea (tak ip nē´ ə)
ureterolithotomy
   (yer rē´ ter ō lith ot´ ō mē)
ureterorrhaphy (yer rē ter ôr´ ə fē)
ureterotomy (yer e throt´ ə mē)
urethralgia (yer ə thral´ jē ə)
urethrotomy (yer ē ter ot´ə mē)

Complete the Unit 4 Self-Test before going on.

Unit 4 Self-Test

PART 1

From the list on the right, select the correct meaning for each of the following terms:

_____ 1.Urethrospasm
_____ 2. Spermatoid
_____ 3. Nephroptosis
_____ 4. Anomaly
_____ 5. Oophoropexy
_____ 6. Bradypnea
_____ 7. Angioblast
_____ 8. Ureterotomy
_____ 9. Angiosclerosis
_____ 10. Hysterotomy
_____ 11. Myospasm
_____ 12. Dyspepsia
_____ 13. Hemolysis
_____ 14. Kinesiology
_____ 15. Aneurysm

a. The study (or science) of motion
b. A condition of hardening of vessels
c. Spasm of the urethra
d. Destruction of blood (cells)
e. Abnormally slow breathing
f. Surgical fixation of the ovary
g. Tumor of nerve and fibrous tissue
h. Muscle spasm
i. Structure contrary to the rule
j. Resembling sperm
k. Abnormally enlarged kidney
l. Ballooning out of blood vessel
m. Painful menstruation (cramps)
n. Embryonic vessel cell
o. Kidney out of its normal place (dropped kidney)
p. Incision into the uterus (cesarean section)
q. Painful digestion (heartburn)
r. Incision into the ureter

PART 2

Complete each of the medical terms on the right with the appropriate missing part:

1. A condition of hardening of muscle _____ sclerosis
2. Kidney stone   Nephro _____
3. Abnormally fast breathing   Tachy _____

4. Painful menstruation   _____ menorrhea

5. Spasm of the uterus   _____ spasm

6. Cessation of menses   A _____

7. Hemorrhage (bleeding) from the bladder   _____ orrhagia

8. Surgical removal of the ovary   _____ ectomy

9. Incision into the ureter (for the purpose of removing a stone)   _____ lithotomy

10. Surgical removal of the fallopian tube   _____ ectomy

11. Drooping of an organ   P _____

12. Muscle pain due to motion   _____ algia

13. Spasm of the vessels   _____ spasm

14. Protrusion of an organ through a cavity wall   H _____

15. Incision into the urethra   _____ otomy

ANSWERS

Part 1

1. c	9. b
2. j	10. p
3. o	11. h
4. i	12. q
5. f	13. d
6. e	14. a
7. n	15. l
8. r	

Part 2

1. Myosclerosis	9. Ureterolithotomy
2. Nephrolith	10. Salpingectomy
3. Tachypnea	11. Ptosis
4. Dysmenorrhea	12. Kinesialgia
5. Hysterospasm	13. Angiospasm
6. Amenorrhea	14. Hernia
7. Cystorrhagia	15. Urethrotomy
8. Oophorectomy	

Unit 5

In this unit, you will form more than 100 new medical terms. Some words will be formed by using parts you already know. You will also use the following new word roots, prefixes, and suffixes:

algesia (*oversensitivity to pain*)
cheil/o (*lip*)
col/o (*colon*)
dactyl/o (*fingers or toes*)
enter/o (*intestine*)
esophag/o (*esophagus*)
esthesia (*feeling, sensation*)
gingiv/o (*gums*)
gloss/o (*tongue*)
hepat/o (*liver*)
ile/o (*ileum*)

jejun/o (*jejunum*)
myel/o (*spinal cord, bone marrow*)
pancreat/o (*pancreas*)
phas/o (*speech*)
phleb/o (*veins*)
plas/o (*formation*)
proct/o (*rectum and anus*)
rect/o (*rectum*)
splen/o (*spleen*)
stomat/o (*mouth*)

dys- (*bad, difficult, painful*)
macro- (*large*)
micro- (*small*)
poly- (*many*)
sym-, syn- (*together*)

-clysis (*irrigation*)
-ectasia (*dilatation, stretching*)
-orrhexis (*rupture, bursting apart*)
-plegia, -plegic (*paralysis*)
-scope, -scopy (*look, examine*)
-tripsy (*crushing*)

Now you'll learn some terms relating to the digestive system. Digestion is the process by which food is broken down mechanically and chemically in the gastrointestinal tract. It is converted into absorbable form. The tissues then synthesize these forms and produce energy.

Refer to the accompanying illustration and the table that follows to work through frames 1 to 32.

The Digestive System

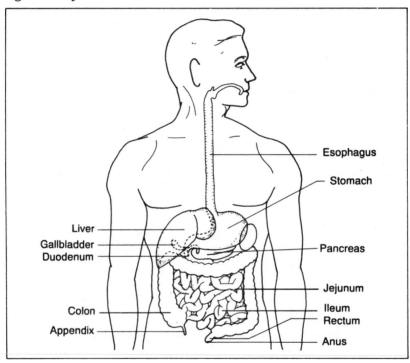

The Digestive System

1.

ORGAN	WORD ROOT FOR ORGAN	ANOTHER WORD ROOT OR COMBINING FORM
mouth	stomat/o	algia—pain
lip	cheil/o	
teeth	dent/o	clysis—washing or irrigation
gums	gingiv/o	(*word in itself*)
tongue	gloss/o	
		plasty—surgical repair
esophagus	esophag/o	(*plastic surgery*)
stomach	gastr/o	cele—herniation
small intestine	enter/o	ectasia—dilatation or
duodenum (1st part)	duoden/o	stretching (*word in itself*)
jejunum (2nd part)	jejun/o	centesis—puncture (or tap) to draw fluid
ileum (3rd part)	ile/o	ptosis—prolapse or drooping
large intestine or colon	col/o	pexy—surgical fixation
		orrhexis—rupture
		orrhagia—hemorrhage
rectum	rect/o	
		orrhaphy—suturing of
anus and rectum	proct/o	

combining form	suffix
scop/o (examine)	y—noun (*process or action*)
	ic—pertaining to
pleg/a (paralysis)	ia—condition
	ic—pertaining to

glands of digestion
  liver   hepat/o
  pancreas   pancreat/o

2.

stomat/o

The word root for mouth is

_____ / __ .

3.

inflammation of
    the mouth

Stomat/itis means _____

_____.

surgical repair of
    the mouth

Stomat/o/plast/y means _____

_____.

4.

stomat/algia
stomatalgia
stō mä tal´ jē ə

Using the word root for mouth, form a word
meaning painful mouth,

_____ / _____ ;

stomat/orrhagia
stomatorrhagia
stō mat´ ō rä´ jē ə

hemorrhage of the mouth,

_____ / _____ .

5.

gloss/o
painful tongue
excision of
    the tongue
spasm or twitching
    of the tongue

Refer to the table. The word root for tongue is

_____ / __ .

Gloss/algia means _____.

Gloss/ectomy means _____

_____ .

Gloss/o/spasm means _____

_____.

6.

gloss/itis
glossitis
glos ī´ tis

Using the word root, build a word meaning
inflammation of the tongue,

_____ / __ ;

gloss/al
glossal
glos´ əl

pertaining to the tongue,

_____ / al __ .

7.

hypo/gloss/al
hypoglossal
hī′ pō glos′ əl

What word would you use to describe a medication that is administered under the tongue?

_____/_____/_____

under   tongue   pertaining to

8.

gloss/o/pleg/ia
glossoplegia
glos ō plē′ jē ə

Using the information needed from the table, build a word meaning paralysis of the tongue (noun),

_____/___/_____/_____;

condition

gloss/o/pleg/ic
glossoplegic
glos ō ple′ jik

paralysis of the tongue,

_____/___/_____/_____.

pertaining to

9.

Go back to the table. The word root for lip is

cheil
cheil/o

_____. The combining form for lip is

_____/___.

10.

inflammation of
the lips

Cheil/itis means _____
_____.

plastic surgery of
the lips

Cheil/o/plast/y means _____
_____.

cheil/otomy
cheilotomy
kē lot′ ō mē

11.

Build a word meaning incision into the lips,

_____/_____;

cheil/osis
cheilosis
kē lō′ sis

abnormal condition or diseased condition of the

lips, _____/_____.

cheil/o/stomat/o/
   plast/y
cheilostomatoplasty
kē´ lō stō mat´ ō
   plas tē

12.
A word meaning plastic surgery of the lips and
mouth is
_____ / _/ _____ / _/ _____ / ___.
    lip   mouth   repair process of

gingiv/o
pertaining to gums

13.
The word root for gums is
_____ / ___. Gingival means
_____.

gingiv/itis
gingivitis
jin ji vī´ tis

gingiv/algia
gingivalgia
jin ji val´ jē ə

gingiv/ectomy
gingivectomy
jin ji vek´ tə mē

gingiv/o/gloss/itis
gingivoglossitis
jin´ ji vō glos ī´ tis

14.
Build a word meaning inflammation of the gums,
_____ / _____;

painful gums,
_____ / _____;

excision of gum tissue,
_____ / _____;

inflammation of the gums and tongue,
_____ / _/ _____ / ____.

stomach
  hemorrhage
inflammation of
  the stomach
pertaining to the
  stomach

15.
Here are some easy ones. Gastr/orrhagia means
_____.
Gastr/itis means _____
_____.
Gastr/ic means _____
_____.

gastr/ectasia
gastrectasia
gas trek tā´ zhə

16.
Go back to the table for help on this one. Form a
word meaning dilatation (stretching) of the
stomach: _____ / _____.

gastr/o/enter/
   ostomy
gastroenterostomy
gas´ trō en ter os´
   tō mē

17.
Form a wording meaning surgical procedure to
form a new opening between the stomach
and small intestine,
_____ / / _____ / _____;

gastr/o/enter/ic
gastroenteric
gas´ trō en ter´ ik

pertaining to the stomach and small intestine,
_____ / / _____ / _____.

enter/o/clysis
enteroclysis
en ter ok´ li sis

18.
Refer to the table again. Build a word meaning
washing or irrigation of the small intestine,
_____ / / _____;

enter/ectasia
enterectasia
en´ ter ek tā´ jē ə

dilatation of the small intestine,
_____ / _____.

poisoning of the
   small intestine
puncture of the
   small intestine
intestinal
   hernia

19.
What do the following terms mean?
Enter/o/toxin _____
_____.

Enter/o/centesis _____
_____.

Enter/o/cele _____
_____.

pertaining to the
   colon or large
   intestine
puncture of the
   colon
making a new open-
   ing into the colon

20.
Try these.
Col/ic _____
_____
_____.

Col/o/centesis _____
_____.

Col/ostomy _____
_____.

col/o/pex/y
colopexy
kō´ lō pek sē

21.
Build a word meaning surgical fixation of the
colon, _____ / / _____ / ___;

col/o/clysis
coloclysis
kō lok´ li sis

washing or irrigation of the colon,
_____ / / _____;

col/itis
colitis
kō lī´ tis

inflammation of the colon,
_____ / _____.

rect/o

22.
Refer to the table again. The word root for rectum is
_____ / ___.

pertaining to the
  rectum

What do each of the following mean?
Rect/al _____
_____.

a rectal
  hernia
washing or
  irrigation of the
  rectum (enema)

Rect/o/cele _____
_____.
Rect/o/clysis _____
_____
_____.

rect/o/urethr/al
rectourethral
rek´ tō yer rēth´ rəl

23.
Build a word meaning pertaining to the rectum and
urethra,
_____ / / _____ / ___;

rect/o/cyst/otomy
rectocystotomy
rek´ tō sis tot´ ə mē

incision of the bladder through the rectum,
_____ / / _____ / ___.
     rectum   bladder   incision

specializes in
  diseases of the
  anus and rectum

24.
Proctology is the study of diseases of the anus and
rectum. A proct/o/log/ ist is one who _____
_____.

25.

proct/o/clysis
proctoclysis
(enema)

Build a word meaning washing or irrigation of anus and rectum,

prok tok´ li sis

_____ / / _____;

proctoplegia or
proctoparalysis

paralysis of the opening from the anus,

_____.

26.

instrument for
examining the
anus and rectum
prok´ tə skōp

Write a meaning for each of the following:

proct/o/scope _____

_____

_____.

examination of the
anus and rectum
prok tos´ kō pē

proct/o/scopy _____

_____.

27.

pertaining to the
liver

Back to the table. Hepat/ic means _____

_____.

enlargement of the
liver

Hepatomegaly means _____

_____.

28.

hepat/o/scop/y
hepatoscopy
hep ə tos´ kō pē

Build a word meaning inspection (examination) of the liver,

_____ / / _____ / __;

hepat/otomy
hepatotomy
hep ə tot´ ō mē

incision into the liver,

_____ / _____;

hepat/itis
hepatitis
hep ə tī´ tis

inflammation of the liver,

_____ / _____.

29.

pertaining to the
pancreas

Here's another new word root. Pancreat/ic means
_____ .

destruction of
pancreatic tissue

Pancreat/o/lys/is means _____
_____ .

30.

pancreat/o/lith
pancreatolith
pan krē at´ ə lith

Build a word meaning a stone or calculus in the
pancreas,
_____/____/_____ ;

pancreas   stone

pancreat/itis
pancreatitis
pan krē a tī´ tis

inflammation of the pancreas,
_____/_____ ;

pancreat/ectomy
pancreatectomy
pan krē a tek´ tō mē

excision of part or all of the pancreas,
_____/_____ ;

pancreat/otomy
pancreatotomy
pan krē a tot´ ə mē

incision into the pancreas,
_____/_____ .

31.

esophag/o/duoden/
ostomy
esophagoduoden-
ostomy
ē sof´ ə gō dōō´ ō
den os´ tō mē

When an entire gastrectomy is performed, a new
connection (opening) is formed between the
esophagus and duodenum. This is called an
_____/____/_____/_____ .
(Note: Remember to name the anatomical parts in
the order in which food passes through them.)

32.
As you rewrite each of the following, analyze it (make your own diagonal divisions) and pronounce it to yourself: gastroenterocolostomy,

gastr/o/enter/o/
  col/ostomy

_____;

esophagogastrostomy,

esophag/o/gastr/
  ostomy

_____;

enterocholecystostomy,

enter/o/chol/e/
  cyst/ostomy

_____.

33.
Try it again:
jejunoileostomy,

jejun/o/ile/
  ostomy

_____;

duodenocholecystostomy,

duoden/o/chol/e/
  cyst/ostomy

_____;

esophagogastroscopy,

esophag/o/gastr/
  o/scopy

_____.

34.
Splen/o is used in words about the spleen. Build a word meaning excision of the spleen,

splen/ectomy
splen ek´ tō mē

_____/_____;

enlargement of the spleen,

splen/o/megal/y
splen´ ō meg ə lē

_____/_____/___;

hemorrhage from the spleen,

splen/orrhagia
splen or ä´ jē ə

_____/_____.

35.
Write a meaning for
splen/algia,

pain in the spleen

_____;

splen/o/hepat/o/megaly,

enlargement of
  both spleen and
  liver

_____;

splen/ic,

pertaining to the
  spleen

_____.

36.

Let's review what you just covered. Using the suggested answers, write the meaning of each of the following terms.

SUGGESTED ANSWERS:

colon	jejunum	rectum
duodenum	lips	rectum and anus
esophagus	liver	small intestine
gums	mouth	tongue
stomach	pancreas	

rectum	rect/o	_____
colon	col/o	_____
pancreas	pancreat/o	_____
rectum and anus	proct/o	_____
lips	cheil/o	_____
mouth	stomat/o	_____
small intestine	enter/o	_____
esophagus	esophag/o	_____
gums	gingiv/o	_____
tongue	gloss/o	_____
jejunum	jejun/o	_____
liver	hepat/o	_____
duodenum	duoden/o	_____
stomach	gastr/o	_____

37.

Try these.

SUGGESTED ANSWERS:

repair (renew)	stretching
paralysis	irrigation

irrigation	-clysis	_____
paralysis	-plegia	_____
repair (renew)	-plasty	_____
stretching	-ectasia	_____

Here's what we suggest:

38.
In your own words, write the meaning of each of the following medical terms.

a new opening between duodenum and jejunum

duoden/o/jejun/ostomy

_____

_____

inspection of the rectum and lower colon (with an instrument)

proct/oscopy

_____

_____

cheil/o/plasty

plastic surgery of the lips

_____

_____

esophag/o/ectasia

stretching of the esophagus

_____

_____

irrigation of the rectum and lower colon (enema)

proct/o/clysis

_____

_____

pain of the stomach and intestine

gastr/o/enter/algia

_____

_____

pancreat/otomy

incision into the pancreas

_____

_____

stomat/oma

tumor of the mouth

_____

_____

gloss/o/plegia

paralysis of the tongue

_____

_____

39.

Let's try something different. Some terms referring to abnormal conditions related to the heart or blood vessels can be confusing. Read each definition carefully and select the terms that refer to a condition or procedure involving only the heart. Put an X in the box.

☐ thrombus

☒ coronary thrombosis

☐ embolus

☐ embolism

☒ cardiac arrest

☒ fibrillation

☒ defibrillation

☐ *Thrombus* is a blood clot.

☐ *Coronary thrombosis* is a heart attack caused by a blood clot that occludes (closes off) a coronary vessel of the heart.

☐ *Embolus* is a foreign or abnormal particle circulating in the blood, such as a bubble of air, a blood clot, or cholesterol plaque.

☐ *Embolism* is the sudden obstruction of a blood vessel by an embolus.

☐ *Cardiac arrest* is the complete cessation of heart function. (If the heartbeat cannot be restored, the patient dies.)

☐ *Fibrillation* means very fast and irregular heartbeat.

☐ *Defibrillation* means using an electrical spark to shock the heart and bring about a slower and regular heartbeat.

Now review the terms and their meanings again. This time *circle* each term that refers to a condition of the blood or blood vessels.

40.

Try these. A blood clot floating through the blood stream is known as a *thrombus*. When a blood clot occludes a vessel, the condition is called *thrombosis*. The part of the word meaning abnormal or diseased condition is

-osis

_____.

41.
An embolus is any foreign or abnormal particle circulating in the blood, such as an air bubble, a cholesterol deposit, or even a blood clot. Embolism is the condition caused by an

embolus
em´ bō lus

_____.

thrombus
throm´ bus

A circulating blood clot is a _____.
But any foreign particle (including a blood clot) circulating through the bloodstream is an

embolus

_____.

42.
When a vessel is suddenly occluded by an embolus, the resulting condition is known as an

embol (ism)
em´ bō lizm

_____ism.

thromb (osis)
throm bō´ sis

When a sudden vessel occlusion is caused by a thrombus, the resulting condition is a
_____osis.

thrombosis

A blood clot occluding a coronary (heart) vessel is a coronary _____.

43.
Embolism is caused by a/an

embolus

_____.

Thrombosis is caused by a/an

thrombus

_____.

44.
A sudden blocking or occlusion of the coronary vessel of the heart by a blood clot is a/an

coronary
    thrombosis

_____.

45.

Cardiac fibrillation may result from coronary thrombosis. The heart beats 200 to 400 times a minute and is very irregular. If something is not done quickly, fibrillation will exhaust the heart and it will stop beating altogether.

defibrillation
dē fĭb ri lā´ shun

Underline the term that indicates the better outcome: cardiac arrest / defibrillation

46.

A very fast, irregular heartbeat, left unchecked, may lead to a complete cessation of heart functioning

cardiac arrest

known as _____.

47.

A very fast, irregular heartbeat is called fibrillation. Using an electrical spark to shock the heart and bring about a regular heartbeat is called

(de)fibrillation

de_____.

48.

Write the correct term for each of the following definitions:

a blood clot floating through the bloodstream,

thrombus

_____;

using an electrical spark to shock the heart and

defibrillation

restore a regular heartbeat, _____;

complete cessation of heart functioning,

cardiac arrest

_____ _____;

a very fast, irregular heartbeat,

fibrillation

_____;

sudden blocking or occlusion of a vessel by something that floated in the bloodstream,

embolism

_____;

sudden blocking of the coronary vessel by a blood clot,

coronary
  thrombosis

_____ _____.

49.
Arteries are vessels that carry blood *away* from the heart. Veins are vessels that carry blood back *to* the

heart   _____.

50.
Note: Angi/o is the term used for vessels, whether the vessel is an artery or a vein.

51.
A word root for vein is phleb/o. If arteriosclerosis is

arteries   hardening of the _____,

phleb/o/scler/osis   then hardening of veins is called
phlebosclerosis
flēb´ ō skler ō´ sis   _____ / ___ / _____ / _____.
                                vein   hardening   condition

52.
phleb/otomy   Build a word meaning incision into a vein
phlebotomy   (venisection or cut down),
flē bot´ ō mē   _____ / _____;

phleb/itis
phlebitis   inflammation of a vein,
flē bī´ tis   _____ / _____.

53.
Thromb/o is the word root that means clot.
Thromb/o/angi/itis means inflammation of a vessel
clot   with formation of a _____.

54.
excision of a   Thromb/ectomy means _____
  thrombus (clot)   _____.

inflammation of a
    vein with
    thrombus
    formation

55.
Thromb/o/phleb/itis means _____

_____

_____.

56.
A synonym for clot is

thrombus

_____.

57.
thromb/osis   Build a word meaning
thrombosis   a condition caused by a clot,
throm bō´ sis   _____/_____;

thromb/o/cyte
thrombocyte   a cell that aids in clotting,
throm´ bō sīt   _____/___/_____;

thromb/oid
thromboid   resembling a clot,
throm´ boid   _____/_____.

58.
Orrhexis is a suffix meaning rupture.
rupture of the   Cyst/orrhexis means _____
    bladder   _____.
rupture of the   Enter/orrhexis means _____
    small intestine _____.
rupture of a blood   Angi/orrhexis means _____
    vessel   _____.

59.
cardi/orrhexis   Build a word meaning
cardiorrhexis   rupture of the heart,
kär dē ō rek´ sis   _____/_____;

phleb/orrhexis
phleborrhexis   rupture of a vein,
flē bō rek´ sis   _____/_____.

60.
Here's a chance to use all the "rrh" suffixes:
-orrhexis, -orrhagia, -orrhaphy, -orrhea. Build a
word meaning:
rupture of the bladder,

cyst/orrhexis _____/_____;

hemorrhage from the liver,

hepat/orrhagia _____/_____;

flowing from the nose ("runny" nose),

rhin/orrhea _____/_____;

suturing (or joining) the fallopian tubes,

salping/orrhaphy _____/_____.

suturing (or closing)   What does herniorrhaphy mean?
 a rupture   _____.

61.
An- is a form of the prefix *a-* meaning without.
Esthesia means feeling or sensation. Give the
meaning of the following words:

a drug that removes   anesthesia _____
 feeling (literally,   _____
 without feeling)   _____;
the study or   anesthesiology _____
 science of   _____
 removing feeling   _____;
instrument for   esthesiometer _____
 measuring feel-   _____
 ing or sensation   _____;
abnormal sensi-   hyperesthesia _____
 tivity (to pain)   _____.

62.
an/esthesi/o/log/ist   Analyze the following words (you do the dividing):
an es thēz ē ol´ ō   anesthesiologist,
 jist   _____;
hypo/esthes/ia   hypoesthesia,
hī pō es thē´ zē ə   _____.

63.

without sensitivity
to pain
an´ al jē´ zē ə

Algesia is a word meaning a sense of pain. What does analgesia mean? _____ _____.

64.

The prefixes *a*- and *an*- mean without. Examine the following two lists of words:

an/*a*lgesia	a/*b*iotic
an/*e*mia	a/*d*ermia
an/*e*ncephalus	a/*f*ebrile
an/*e*sthesia	a/*k*inesia
an/*o*nychia	a/*m*enia
an/*o*pia	a/*m*enorrhea
an/*u*ria	a/*p*nea
an/*u*resis	a/*s*epsis

Draw a conclusion: When the word root begins with a consonant, use the prefix _____.

a-

an-

When the word root begins with a vowel, use the prefix _____.

65.

Put the proper form of the prefix before each of the following roots and then write a meaning for each.

anemic—a
  condition of less
  blood
astomia—without a
  mouth
  (congenital)
afebrile—without
  fever
anodontia—
  toothless

_____emic _____ _____;

_____stomia _____ _____;

_____febrile _____;

_____odontia _____.

66.
Here's some practice with other prefixes. Phas/o means speech. Write a meaning for each of the following:

speechless   aphasia _____;

abnormally fast
   speech   tachyphasia _____
            _____;
abnormally slow
   speech   bradyphasia _____
            _____;
pain or difficulty
   when speaking   dysphasia _____
            _____.

67.
pain along the
   course of a nerve
   (or equivalent)   Neur/o is used in words that refer to nerves.
            Neur/algia means _____
            _____.

68.
Tripsis, from which we get trips/y, is a Greek word that means "rub" or "massage." Neur/o/trips/y means surgical crushing of a nerve. The word root for crushing (usually by rubbing or grinding) is

trips   _____.

neur/o/trips/y   Tripsis can be carried to the point of crushing or
neurotripsy   grinding. Surgical crushing of a nerve is called
nyōō′ rō trip sē   _____ / ____ / _____ / ____.

69.
In some cases of lithiasis, it may be necessary to
lith/o/trips/y   crush calculi so they can pass. A word meaning
lithotripsy   surgical crushing of stones is
lith′ ō trip sē   _____ / ____ / _____ / ____.

70.
Myel/itis can mean either inflammation of bone
marrow or inflammation of the spinal cord. From
the definitions, you may conclude that myel is

bone marrow
spinal cord

the word root for both _____ and

_____ .

71.
The suffix o/blast means embryonic (germ), or a
cell giving rise to something else. In the word
myel/o/blast, the word root myel refers to bone

bone marrow
  germinating cell

marrow. Write the meaning of myel/o/blast:

_____ .

In myel/o/cele, the word root refers to spinal cord.

hernia of the spinal
  cord

Write the meaning of myel/o/cele: _____

_____ .

72.
You have learned that dys- means pain, painful.
But dys- is a prefix that also means bad (defective)
or difficult. Try the next few examples.

73.
Plas/ia or plas/is means formation or change in the
sense of molding. This kind of formation occurs

bad, defective
  (poor or
  abnormal
  formation)

naturally instead of being done by a plastic
surgeon. Dys/plas/ia means _____

_____

_____ .

74.
A/plas/ia means failure of an organ to develop

hyper/plas/ia
hyperplasia
hī´ per plā´ zha

properly. A word that means overgrowth or too
much development is

_____ / _____ / _____ .

75.
hypo/plas/ia
hypoplasia   If overdevelopment is hyperplasia,
hī´ pō plā´ zha   underdevelopment is expressed as

_____ / _____ / ____.

chondr/o/dys/   76.
    plas/ia   Myel/o/dys/plas/ia means defective
chondrodysplasia   development of the spinal cord. What does
kon´ drō dis plā´ zha   chondr/o/dys/plas/ia mean? _____
bad (defective)   _____
    development of _____.
    cartilage

oste/o/chondr/o/   77.
    dys/plas/ia   Write the meaning of osteochondrodysplasia. _____
osteochondrodys-   _____
    plasia   _____.
os´ tē ō kon´ drō dis
    plā´ zhə
defective formation
    of bone and
    cartilage

                    78.
                    The micron (1/1000 mm) is a unit of measurement.
microns   Many cocci are 2 microns in diameter. A red blood
mī´ krons   cell is 7 _____ in diameter.

micr/o/meter   An instrument for measuring the diameter of
micrometer   something microscopic is a
mī krom´ ə ter   _____ / ___ / _____.

                    79.
                    Macr/o is the opposite of micr/o. Macr/o is used in
large   words to mean _____.

80.
Things that are macr/o/scop/ic can be seen with the naked eye. Give a meaning for macroblast.

a large embryonic
(or germ) cell

_____

_____ .

81.

Macr/o/cephal/us
mak rō se fal´ us

An abnormally large head is

_____ / ___ / _____ / ___ .

macr/o/cyte

An abnormally large cell is a

_____ / ___ / _____ .

macr/o/cocc/us

A very large coccus is called a

_____ / ___ / _____ / ___ .

82.

abnormally large
tongue

Macr/o/gloss/ia means _____

_____ .

abnormally large
ear(s)

Macr/ot/ia means _____

_____ .

abnormally large
nose

Macr/o/rhin/ia means _____

_____ .

abnormally large
lips
mak rō kē´ lē ə

Macr/o/cheil/ia means _____

_____ .

83.
Macr/o/dactyl/ia means abnormally large fingers

dactyl
dak´ til

or toes. The word root for fingers or toes is

_____ .

englarged digits, or
another way of
saying large
fingers or toes

84.
What does dactyl/o/megal/y mean? _____

_____ .

85.

dactyl or
dactyl/o

A finger or toe is called a digit. But the root for digit is _____/_____.

dactyl/itis
dactylitis
dak til ī´ tis

Build a word meaning
inflammation of a digit,
_____/_____;

dactyl/o/spasm
dactylospasm
dak til´ ō spa zm

cramp or spasm of a digit,
_____/____/_____;

dactyl/o/gram
dactylogram
dak til´ ō gram

a fingerprint,
_____/____/_____.

abnormally large
   fingers and toes
   (digits)
fingers or toes
   (digits)

86.
Macr/o/dactyl/ia means _____
_____.
Poly/dactyl/ism means too many _____
_____.

87.
Poly- is a prefix meaning too many or too much.
Poly/ur/ia means excessive amount of urine. When a person drinks a lot of fluid,
_____/_____/_____ results.

poly/ur/ia
polyuria
pol ē yer´ ē ə

88.
Poly/neur/o/path/y means disease of many nerves.

What does poly/neur/itis mean? _____
_____.

polyneuritis
pol ē nyo͞o rī´ tis
inflammation of
   many nerves

89.
Write the meaning of the following:

inflammation of
many joints

Poly/arthr/itis _____

_____;

pain in several
nerves

Poly/neur/algia _____

_____.

90.

syn/ergetic
synergetic
sin er je´ tik

Syn/ergetic means working together. Drugs that
work together to increase the effects of one another
are called _____/_____ drugs.

91.

synergetic

Synergetic muscles are muscles that work together.
Three muscles work together to flex the forearm.
These muscles are _____.

92.

synergetic

APC tablets are thought by some to be more
effective for killing pain than aspirin alone. This is
because *a*spirin, *p*henacetin, and *c*affeine are
_____ drugs.

93.

syn/arth/ro/sis
synarthrosis
a fused joint that
moves as one

Syn/arthr/osis means an immovable joint;
adjoining bones are fused together. When bones of
a joint are fused so they all move as one, the
condition is syn/arthr/osis. What does it mean?

_____.

syndactylism
synarthrosis

Underline the part of the word that means joined
together as one: syndactylism
                      synarthrosis

94.

a condition of two
or more digits
joined together

What does syn/dactyl/ism mean (-ism denotes a
medical condition or disease)? _____

_____.

95.

together or joined
as one

Syn- and sym- are different forms of the same
prefix: Syn- and sym- mean _____

_____.

96.

Use the prefix sym- when the word root begins
with the consonants b, m, or p; use syn- in all other
cases. Write the prefix for each of the following:

synarthrosis   _____ arthrosis
symmetrical   _____ metrical
symbolism   _____ bolism
symphysis   _____ physis
syndrome   _____ drome
sympathy   _____ pathy
symbiosis   _____ biosis

97.

joined as one,
   together
b, m, p

Both syn- and sym- mean _____
_____; sym- is used when followed by the
letters _____, _____, and _____; syn- is used in
other medical words.

98.

Time to review. Complete each brief definition. Refer to the suggested answers. Write your selection in the space provided.

SUGGESTED ANSWERS:

algesia	phas/o
dactyl/o	phleb/o
embolus	plas/o
esthesia	

esthesia
phleb/o
embolus
algesia
phas/o
plas/o
dactyl/o

oversensitivity to pain _____

veins _____

circulating foreign particle _____

feeling, sensation _____

speech _____

formation, development _____

digits _____

99.

Try these.

SUGGESTED ANSWERS:

a-, an-	-orrhagia
dys-	-orrhaphy
macro-	-orrhexis
micro-	syn-, sym-
-orrhea	-tripsy

-orrhexis
syn-, sym-
dys-
-orrhagia
macro-
-tripsy
micro-
-orrhea
a-, an-
-orrhaphy

rupture _____

together _____

defective, difficult, painful _____

hemorrhage _____

large _____

crushing _____

microscopic _____

flowing forth _____

without _____

suturing (repair of) _____

Here are some suggestions:	100. In your own words, write the meaning for each of the following:
crushing of a nerve	neur/o/tripsy _____
without sensation	an/esthesia _____
bad formation of the spinal cord	myel/o/dys/plasia _____
a condition of a blood clot in the coronary artery	coronary thrombosis _____
pertaining to something too small to see with the naked eye	micro/scop/ic _____
speechless	a/phasia _____
a condition of fingers joined together	syn/dactyl/ism _____
surgical repair of a hernia	herni/orrhaphy _____
hemorrhage of the liver	hepat/orrhagia _____
without pain	an/algesia _____
complete cessation of heart function	cardiac arrest _____
electrical shock of the heart to restore regular rhythm	defibrillation _____
ruptured blood vessel	phleb/orrhexis _____

101.

Here are 50 medical terms for practicing your pronunciation. Say the term aloud and then say what it means. Then take the Unit 5 Self-Test.

analgesia (an´ al jē´zē ə)

anesthesiologist
   (an´ es thē zē ol´ ō jist)

angiogram (an´ gē ō gram)

cardiorrhexis (kär dē ōr rek´ sis)

cheilitis (kē lī´ tis)

cheiloplasty (kē´ lō plas tē)

chondrodysplasia
   (kon´ drō dis plā´ zhə)

colic (kol´ ik)

colitis (kō lī´ tis)

colostomy (kō los´ tō mē)

cystorrhexis (sis tō rek´ sis)

dactylogram (dak til´ ō gram)

dactylomegaly
   (dak´ til ō meg´ ə lē)

defibrillation (dē fib ri lā´ shun)

embolism (em´bō lizm)

embolus (em´ bō lus)

enterocele (en´ ter ō sēl)

enteroclysis (en ter ok´ li sis)

esophagogastroscopy
   (ē sof´ ə gō gas tros´ kō pē)

esthesiometer (es thē zē om´ ə ter)

gastrectasia (gas trek tā´ zhə)

gastrorrhagia (gas´ trō rä´ jē ə)

gingivoglossitis
   (jin´ ji vō glos ī´ tis)

glossoplegia (glos ō plē´ jē ə)

hepatitis (hep a tī´ tis)

hepatomegaly (hep a tō meg´ a lē)

hepatorrhagia (hep a tō rä´ jē a)

hyperesthesia (hī´ per es thē´ zhə)

hypoesthesia (hī´ pō es thē´ zhə)

hypoglossal (hī´ pō glos´ əl)

hysterorrhexis (his´ ter ō rek´ sis)

ileoplegia (il ē ō plā jē ə)

jejunoileostomy
   (je ju´ nō il ē os´ tō mē)

lithotripsy (lith´ ō trip sē)

macrocephalus
   (mak´ rō se fal´ us)

macrocheilia (mak´ rō kē´ lē ə)

micrometer (mī krom´ ə ter)

neuromyelitis
   (nyōō´ rō mī il ī´ tis)

neurotripsy (nyōō´ rō trip sē)

pancreatectomy
   (pan krē a tek´ tō mē)

phlebitis (flē bī´ tis)

polyarthritis (pol ē arth rī´ tis)

polyuria (pol ē yer´ ē ə)

proctoclysis (prok tok´ li sis)

proctoscopy (prok tos´ kō pē)

rectal (rek´ t'l)

syndactylism (sin dak´ til izm)

stomatitis (stō mä tī´ tis)

thrombosis (throm bō´ sis)

thrombus (throm´ bus)

Unit 5 Self-Test

PART 1

From the list on the right, select the correct meaning for each of the following often used medical terms.

_____ 1. Lithotripsy
_____ 2. Thrombosis
_____ 3. Polyarthritis
_____ 4. Anesthetist
_____ 5. Colic
_____ 6. Phlebitis
_____ 7. Glossoplegia
_____ 8. Dactylogram
_____ 9. Analgesia
_____ 10. Cheilitis
_____ 11. Neuromyelitis
_____ 12. Macrocephalus
_____ 13. Hypoesthesia
_____ 14. Hepatomegaly
_____ 15. Aphasia

a. Inflammation of the vein
b. Abnormal enlargement of the liver
c. Crushing (destruction) of a nerve
d. Paralysis of the tongue
e. Abnormally enlarged head
f. Absence of pain
g. Inflammation of many joints
h. Under the tongue (sublingual)
i. A specialist who removes the sensation of pain
j. Crushing of a calculus
k. Relating to the colon
l. Fingerprint
m. Speechless
n. Clotted condition of a blood vessel
o. Inflammation of the nerves of the spinal cord
p. Less than normal sensation
q. Inflammation of the lips

PART 2

Complete each of the medical terms on the right with the appropriate missing part. Some terms are missing all parts!

1. Rupture of the bladder   _____ orrhexis
2. Abnormally intense feeling or
   sensation (pain)   _____ esthesia
3. Foreign particle occluding a
   small blood vessel   _____ ism

4. Rupture of the heart   _____

5. Abnormally enlarged lips   Macro _____

6. Stretching or dilatation of the
   stomach   _____ ectasia

7. Paralysis of the ileum   Ileo _____

8. Stopped heart   _____ (two words)

9. Abnormally enlarged fingers   Dactylo _____

10. Inflammation of the liver   _____

11. Instrument for measuring
    sensation   _____ meter

12. Pertaining to the rectum   _____

13. Formation of a new opening
    in the colon   _____

14. Painful tongue   _____

15. Growing together of fingers
    and toes   _____ ism

ANSWERS

Part 1

1. j	9. f
2. n	10. q
3. g	11. o
4. i	12. e
5. k	13. p
6. a	14. b
7. d	15. m
8. l	

Part 2

1. Cystorrhexis	9. Dactylomegaly
2. Hyperesthesia	10. Hepatitis
3. Embolism	11. Esthesiometer
4. Cardiorrhexis	12. Rectal
5. Macrocheilia	13. Colostomy
6. Gastrectasia	14. Glossalgia
7. Ileoplegia	15. Syndactylism
8. Cardiac arrest	

Unit 6

In this unit you will learn many terms related to symptoms, diagnoses, treatments, and statistics. Some words will be familiar, but you'll use them in new ways.

<u>Signs</u>
atrophy
edema
hypertrophy
pulse
respiration
temperature

<u>Symptoms</u>
anorexia
dyspnea
malaise
nausea
tinnitus
vertigo

<u>Qualifiers</u>
acute
central
chronic
generalized
localized
paroxysmal
peripheral

<u>Treatments</u>
active
palliative
prophylactic
systemic

<u>Word Parts</u>
anti- (*against*)
chlor/o (*green*)
erythr/o (*red*)
melan/o (*black*)
pyret/o (*fever*)
xanth/o (*yellow*)

<u>Diagnosis</u>
prodrome
prognosis
syndrome

<u>Statistics</u>
morbidity
mortality

Signs and Symptoms

1.

What is a sign or a symptom? Let's take them one at a time. A sign is any abnormality of the body a physician may discover on examination of the patient. A symptom is also evidence of an abnormality in structure or function. However, the patient experiences a symptom through one or more of the five organs of sense. Can you name them?

sight
sound
smell
taste
feel

_____ _____ _____ _____ _____

2.

Simply put, a sign or a symptom is evidence there is something wrong. The patient feels, tastes, or hears something that is out of the ordinary and tells the examiner about it. This symptomatic evidence may not be apparent to the examiner. On the other hand, sometimes evidence can be observed by the examiner and also be experienced by the patient. Check the box that indicates whether the evidence described is a sign, a symptom, or both.

	sign	symptom	both	
both	☐	☐	☐	swelling of the wrist
symptom	☐	☐	☐	ringing (tinkling sound) in the ear
symptom	☐	☐	☐	sourness in the mouth
symptom	☐	☐	☐	ammonia sensation in the nose
both	☐	☐	☐	painful and swollen elbow
both	☐	☐	☐	bleeding from the nose
both	☐	☐	☐	blue discoloration around the eye
both	☐	☐	☐	very rapid breathing
symptom	☐	☐	☐	pain in the heel
both	☐	☐	☐	chills and fever
both	☐	☐	☐	painful muscle spasm in the leg
both	☐	☐	☐	chills, coughing, and runny nose
sign	☐	☐	☐	slow heartbeat
sign	☐	☐	☐	pale complexion
sign	☐	☐	☐	eyes closed, not responding to questions or poking

3.

An abnormality apparent to an examiner
(and sometimes to the patient) is called a

sign   _____.

4.

Any change in body function or structure that the
patient sees, hears, tastes, smells, or feels (and may
not be apparent to an observer) is called a

symptom   _____.

As you can see, most evidence of illness can be
observed by someone other than the patient and
may be experienced by the patient as well.

Vital Signs

5.

Vital means relating to life. A vital sign is evidence
a patient is alive. Body temperature, pulse rate, and
rate of respiration are vital signs because they
provide continuous information about the essential
processes of the body. If one of these signs is
absent, the patient is dead (or in big trouble). Body
temperature, pulse, and respiration are very
important indicators and are called

vital signs   _____.

6

Vital signs can be measured. Temperature (T)
loosely refers to body heat above normal. Normal
body temperature is 98.6°F. Body temperature
increases in a hot environment and during physical
exercise. Many diseases, serious and not serious,
cause a patient's temperature to rise. Elevated body
temperature is called fever. Low fever is 99° to
101°F. Moderate fever is 101° to 103°F. High fever
is 103° to 105°F. A patient who is afebrile has a
normal body temperature, which is approximately

98.6   _____ °F.

7.
Pyro is a word root meaning fire or heat.
(Remember the funeral pyres on which the Greeks
and Romans burned their dead?) A pyromaniac has
a fondness for watching things burn or starting

fires   _____.

8.
Pyret/o forms words meaning fever. A patient
described as pyretic would have a temperature

above   _____98.6°F.
                    (above / below / same as)

9.
Pyrexia means feverish. Fever is one way the
body shows something is wrong. Fever can be
observed and measured; therefore, pyrexia is a

sign   _____ of disease.
                        sign / symptom

10.
Hypo/thermia refers to body temperature below
normal. A patient's temperature may be lowered
safely to about 80° during surgery. This controlled
procedure reduces the patient's need for oxygen
and makes some surgical procedures safer. The
hypothermia   patient's lower body temperature is called
hī pō ther´ mē ə
                    _____.

11.
On the other hand, a person who falls through
the ice on a pond in January will surely develop a
life-threatening condition also called

hypothermia   _____.

12.
Injury and dehydration can cause a patient's temperature to rise above 106°F. This life-threatening high temperature is known as _____pyrexia.
(hyper / hypo)

hyper
hī per

13.
In Unit 3 you learned that gen/o means to produce or originate. What does pyret/o/gen mean?
_____.

that which
  produces fever

14.
The measles virus produces fever. Therefore, the virus that causes measles is a
_____.

pyretogen
pī ret´ō jen

15.
Pyret/ic means pertaining to fever. What does pyret/o/gen/ic mean? _____
_____.

pertains to
  something that
  produces fever

16.
Anti- means against. Aspirin is an anti/pyret/ic agent. What does antipyretic mean? _____
_____.

an agent that works
  against fever

17.
Lysis means dissolution or reduction. What does pyret/o/lysis mean? _____.

fever reduction

18.
A physician writes on a patient's chart, "The patient has a low grade fever but is otherwise asymptomatic." What does asymptomatic mean?
_____.

without symptoms

19.

Now let's talk about another vital sign. Pulse (P) is a rhythmical throbbing of the arterial walls. This throbbing is produced when the heart contracts and forces an increased volume of blood into the vessels. After chasing your dog down the street, you would expect your pulse rate to

increase   _____.
                (increase / decrease)

20.

The normal pulse of an average adult is 70 to 80 beats per minute. Fever usually causes a patient's heart to beat more rapidly. When a patient's pulse is 100 beats per minute or higher the condition is

tachycardia   known as _____.
                (tachycardia / bradycardia)
                On the other hand, a pulse less than 60 beats per

bradycardia   minute indicates _____.

21.

The patient usually does not feel a rapid, slow, or irregular pulse. However, a physician can observe and measure pulse rate; therefore, it is said to be a

sign   _____.
                (sign / symptom)

22.

Pulse rate depends on size, sex, age, and physical condition. It's higher in women than men. It's higher in children than adults. But we can say that a healthy adult has an average pulse of (Check one.)
                ☐ 30 to 50 beats per minute.
70 to 80   ☐ 70 to 80 beats per minute.

23.
The pulse is usually felt over the radial artery at the wrist. Although pulse is a simple measure, it provides important evidence about the life (and death) status of the patient. Therefore, it is

vital sign

considered a _____ _____.

24.
Periphery means outer surface of the body.
It is the part of the body away from the center.
A pulse taken at the wrist or ankle is a

peripheral
per i´ fer al

_____ pulse.
(central / peripheral)

25.
A pulse taken near the center of the body, where the heart is, is a _____ pulse.

central

(central / peripheral)

26.

because it is near
   the center of the
   body

A pulse taken with a stethoscope on the chest is a central pulse. Why? _____
_____.

near the outer
   surface of the
   body

27.
What does peripheral mean? _____
_____.

28.
Here's the third vital sign. Respiration (R) is breathing. Breathing is a function of the respiratory system. A breath draws in oxygen. The circulating blood carries the oxygen to the tissues and then returns carbon dioxide to the lungs. The lungs breathe out the waste products of carbon dioxide and water. The normal rate of respiration for an adult is 16 to 18 breaths per minute. A respiration rate of more than 25 breaths per minute is
_____ respiration.

accelerated

(accelerated / decelerated)

29.

an instrument for
measuring
breathing

Pne/o (pronounced nē o) means breath or
breathing. Pne/o/dynamics means the mechanism
of breathing. What does pne/o/meter mean?

_____.

30.

Here's a rule that will help you pronounce words
containing the root pne/o, pne/a. When pne/o
begins the word, the letter "p" is silent. The letter
"p" is pronounced when a prefix comes before it.
Pronounce each of the following:

a/pnea	pronounce: ap´ nē ə
hyper/pnea	pronounce: hī perp´ nē ə
tachy/pnea	pronounce: tak ip nē´ ə
brady/pnea	pronounce: brad´ ip nē ə
pneumon/ia	pronounce: nū mon´ ē ə

31.

very slow
breathing

Bradycardia means very slow heartbeat. What does
brady/pnea mean? _____

_____.

disp´ nē ə
painful (bad)
breathing

32.

Pronounce dys/pnea. What does it mean? _____

_____.

excessively rapid
breathing
hī perp´ nē ə

33.

Hyperpyrexia means excessively high temperature
(over 106°F). What does hyperpnea mean?

_____.

without breathing
ap´ nē ə

34.

A/symptomatic means without symptoms. What
does a/pnea mean? _____.
(Pronounce it.)

35.
Fever and disorders of the lungs or heart may accelerate respiration. Build a word that describes a respiration rate over 25 breaths per minute:

hyperpnea
hī perp´ nē ə

_____.

36.
Very slow breathing of 8 to 9 breaths per minute occurs in serious illnesses like uremia, diabetic coma, and opium poisoning. Build a term that means very slow breathing:

bradypnea
brad ip nē´ ə

_____.

37.
A foreboding irregular and unusual pattern of breathing is called Cheyne-Stokes respiration. (Pronounce *chain-stokes*. It's a condition named after two physicians who first described it more than 150 years ago.) Respiration gradually increases in rapidity and volume until the rate reaches a climax (perhaps 60 to 80 breaths per minute). Then breathing subsides and ceases entirely for up to one minute—when respirations begin again. This condition is due to disturbance of the respiratory center in the brain. It is usually a forerunner of death—but may last several months, days, or even disappear.

38.
Cheyne-Stokes respiration is cyclical. The phase of respiration, at 60 to 80 breaths per minute, is called hyperpnea. What term describes the period when all respiration ceases? _____.

apnea
ap´ nē ə

39.
In certain very serious illnesses, an irregular and arrythmic type of breathing may occur, characterized by both hyperpneic and apneic phases, usually followed by death. It is called

Cheyne-Stokes

C_____-S_____ respiration.

40.
Something is very wrong with the body when a
patient's respiration rate exceeds 25 breaths per
minute. Respiration rate (R), fever (T), and a rapid
pulse (P) are measurable signs of disease. They
indicate the status of the whole body and are

vital signs   called _____ _____

41.

temperature   The vital signs are T _____,
pulse   P _____, and
respiration   R _____.

42.
Let's review. Select the best meaning from column
B for each brief definition in column A. Write your
selection in the space provided.

	Column A	Column B
	bodily change a patient perceives	asymptomatic
symptom	_____	vital signs
see, hear, smell,	sensory ways symptoms are perceived	hyperpyrexia
taste, feel	_____	hypothermia
	temperature, pulse, and respiration	pyretogen
vital signs	_____ _____	pyrteolysis
pyrexia	elevated temperature, fever	pyrexia
pī rek´ sē ə	_____	see, hear,
hypothermia	subnormal body temperature	smell,
hī pō ther´ mē ə	_____	taste, feel
hyperpyrexia	temperature over 106°F	symptom
hī per pī rek´ sē ə	_____	
pyretogen	something that produces fever	
pī ret´ ō gen	_____	
pyretolysis	reduction, dissolution of fever	
pī ret ō lī´ sis	_____	
asymptomatic	lack of symptoms	
ā simp tō mat´ ik	_____	

43.
Now try these.

pulse

peripheral

pne/o, pne/a

bradypnea

dyspnea

hyperpnea

respiration

apnea

Cheyne-Stokes
respiration

	Column A	Column B
	throbbing of an artery in time with the heartbeat	apnea
		bradypnea
	_____	Cheyne-
	pulse taken at the surface of the body	Stokes
	_____	respiration
	two word roots for breath, breathing	dyspnea
	_____ or _____	hyperpnea
	very slow breathing	peripheral
	_____	pne/o, pne/a
	difficult breathing	pulse
	_____	respiration
	excessively fast breathing	
	_____	
	another word for breathing	
	_____	
	respiratory arrest, not breathing	
	_____	
	breathing that reaches a climax, then ceases before beginning again	
	_____ - _____	
	_____	

Color and Other Signs

44.
Color and changes in color of various parts of the body also tell the physician a lot about the patient's condition. Use the information here to build words involving color.

leuk/o	white
melan/o	black
erythr/o	red
cyan/o	blue
chlor/o	green
xanth/o	yellow

45.

xanth/opsia
zan thop´ sē ə
chlor/opia
klor ō´ pē ə

Cyan/opia means blue vision. Form a word meaning

yellow vision, _____/opsia.
green vision, _____/opia.

46.

erythr/o/derma
e rith´ rō der´ mä
melan/o/derma
mel´ a nō der´ mä

Cyan/o/derma means blue skin. Build a word meaning

red skin, _____/__/_____.
black (discolored) skin, _____.

(You draw the lines.)

47.

green (plant) cell
white (blood) cell
red (blood) cell

Write a meaning for each of the following:

chlor/o/cyte, _____.
leuk/o/cyte, _____.
erythr/o/cyte, _____.

48.

melan/o/blast
mel´ a nō blast
erythr/o/blast
e rith´ rō blast

Blast means embryonic cell. Build a word meaning an embryonic cell of the following colors:

embryonic black cell, _____/__/_____.
                            black   embryonic cell
embryonic red cell, _____/__/_____.

49.

a black cell
  carcinoma

Melan/osis means a condition of black pigmentation. Carcinoma is a malignant tumor. What is a melanocarcinoma? _____
_____.

50.

melanocarcinoma
mel´ a nō kär si nō´
  mä

Whenever a hairless mole on the skin turns black and grows larger, a physician should be consulted because there is danger of black mole cancer, or
_____.

51.

green   Chlor/o means _____.

red   Erythr/o means _____.

yellow   Xanth/o means _____.

white   Leuk/o means _____.

Qualifiers

52.

In medical terminology we often use qualifiers. These are adjectives or adverbs that when used with another word make the meaning of that term more specific. Here are a few frequently used qualifiers. Local means a small area or part of the body. General means involving the whole body or many different areas or parts of the body at the same time.

53.

Anesthesia may be considered either local or general. Before extracting a tooth, the dentist injects Novocain to prevent pain. Novocain is a

local   _____ anesthetic.

(local / general)

54.

On the other hand, laughing gas, which puts the

general   patient to sleep, is a _____ anesthetic.

(local / general)

55.
Label each of the following as local or general.
skin rash around the neck and ears,

local
_____.

measles macules from stem to stern,

general
_____.

acne all over the face,

local
_____.

second-degree scalding burn over the belly and

local (two places)   upper thigh, _____.
reddish purple spots over the trunk of the body and
wherever clothing covers the skin,

general
_____.

56.

a small area or part   A localized condition means _____
of the body   _____.
involving the   When a condition is generalized, it means _____
whole body or   _____
many areas at   _____.
the same time

57.
Systemic means pertaining to all body systems, or
the whole body rather than one of its parts. It is
general   another word for _____.
(local/general)

58.
An antihistamine tablet helps a patient breathe
more easily by drying up mucous membranes
inside the nose and sinuses. An antihistamine also
dries up mucous membranes that line all body
systemic   cavities. We say it has a _____
sis tem´ ik   effect.

Other Signs

Besides observing color and color changes, a physician inspects the patient carefully for signs and symptoms that will aid in learning about a patient's disease. Here are some observable changes in the body.

59.
Edema refers to fluid in the tissues. It is a condition in which body tissues accumulate excessive

fluid   _____.

60.
Fluid in the tissues may be local or general. Localized edema involves a small area of the body; generalized edema involves

the whole body   _____.

61.
A bee sting produces an accumulation of fluid in the tissues at the bite site. This is called localized

edema
e dē´ ma   _____.

62.
Heart failure causes severe disturbance of the body's water balance mechanisms. Excessive fluid may accumulate in the lungs, legs, and abdomen.

generalized edema   This is called _____.
                                    (localized/generalized)

63.
Excessive accumulation of fluid in the body tissues

edema   is called _____.

64.

Atrophy is another observable sign of disease. It means a wasting away, or shrinking of tissues, an organ, or the whole body. Underline the word root meaning development.

Atrophy
at´ rō fē

Atrophy

65.

overdevelopment

What does hyper/troph/y mean?

_____ .

Subjective Symptoms

66.

Objective signs such as T, P, and R are signs of primary importance in the investigation of an illness. However, the patient's own concerns and impressions also provide valuable information. Changes in the body not apparent to an observer but experienced by the patient are called symptoms.

67.

Nausea means sickness of the stomach with a desire to vomit. Since it is an internal feeling evident only to the patient, we call it a

symptom

_____ .

68.

nausea
naw´ zē ə

Pain, noxious odors, fevers, and some drugs may cause a sickness of the stomach with a desire to vomit, which is called _____ .

69.
Mal de mer is the French term meaning motion sickness. It is another way to describe the sick feeling of _____.

nausea

70.
Emesis means vomitus—that which is vomited. An irritation of the vomiting center in the brain produces nausea. As a result, the patient ejects the stomach contents through the mouth. The product of vomiting is _____.

emesis (or vomitus)
em´ e sis

71.
Food poisoning, drugs, and fevers can irritate the vomiting center and thus induce _____. The product of vomiting is _____.

vomiting
emesis

72.
Chol/emesis means bile in the vomitus. What does hemat/emesis mean? _____ _____.

blood in the
   vomitus

73.
In an emergency, there are two quick ways to empty the stomach of its contents: (a) use a tube to "pump" the stomach, or (b) give the patient an emetic. What is an emetic? _____ _____.

pertaining to
   something that
   induces
   vomiting

74.
Nausea usually precedes *emesis*. Circle the term that is a subjective symptom. Why? _____ _____.

nausea; the patient
   feels the
   sensation (not
   observable)

75.
In a wide variety of illnesses, two symptoms often occur together. We'll take them one at a time.

malaise

Malaise is a French word literally meaning ill at ease. Underline the part of the word meaning ill.

76.
A patient with infectious mononucleosis may experience a vague sensation of not feeling well, or feeling ill at ease. The symptom is called

malaise
ma lāź

_____.

77.
Malaise is a symptom because the physician cannot observe malaise and does not experience the patient's sensation. Describe malaise. _____

the vague sensation
of not feeling
well

_____.

78.
Orexia means appetite. What does an/orexia mean?

without an appetite
an o rek´ sē ə

_____.

79.
Orexi/mania means an abnormal desire (madness) for food or an uncontrollable appetite. What does orexi/genic mean? _____

pertaining to
  something that
  produces or
  stimulates an
  appetite

_____.

80.
Food that smells good and is appealing to the eye stimulates appetite. We may describe this food and its presentation as _____.

orexigenic
ō reks i gen´ ik

81.
Along with malaise, loss of appetite is a very
common symptom in many diseases. Write the
term for loss of appetite. _____.

anorexia
an o rek´ sē ə

82.
Complete each of the following definitions:
A vague sensation of not feeling well is

malaise
_____.
Sickness of the stomach with a desire to vomit is

nausea
_____.
Another word for vomitus is

emesis
_____.
Elevated body temperature is

pyrexia
_____.
anorexia
Loss of appetite is _____.

83.
A patient with an infection may experience a vague
sensation of not feeling well. A patient with a fever
may not have an appetite. When a fever and
infection occur at the same time, the patient
usually reports these two very subjective
malaise
symptoms. What are they? _____
anorexia
and _____.

84.
the patient
Anorexia and malaise are purely subjective
experiences the
symptoms. What does that mean? _____
sensation
_____.

85.
Vertigo means a turning around. The patient
experiences the sensation of turning around in
space or having objects move about him.

86.
Vertigo is *not* dizziness, faintness, or lightheadedness. However, the patient may have difficulty maintaining equilibrium, and may describe a sensation of spinning or

turning around

_____ in space.

87.
An infection in the middle ear can cause a patient to experience the sensation of turning around in space or of objects moving about her.

symptom
vertigo
ver´ ti gō

This _____ is known as
             (sign/symptom)

_____.

88.
Tinnitus is a jingling, or tinkling, sound in the ear. It is often called ringing in the ear.

tinnitus
ti nī´ tus

Toxicity or sensitivity to a drug like aspirin can cause ringing in the ear. Write the medical term for tinkling sound in the ear: _____.

89.
Ménière's syndrome (pronounce ma nē ars´) is a recurrent and usually progressive group of symptoms including hearing loss, ringing in the ears, a sensation of fullness or pressure in the ears, and a turning around in space.
The term for ringing in the ears is

tinnitus

_____.

The sensation of turning about in space is

vertigo

_____.

90.

Try these and see how much you've learned. Select the best word from the suggested answers.

SUGGESTED ANSWERS:

erythroderma	leukocyte
melanoblast	cyanemia
chlorocyte	xanthemia

chlorocyte
xanthemia
melanoblast
erythroderma
leukocyte
cyanemia

green (plant) cell, _____.
yellowish blood, _____.
black (dark) embryonic cell, _____.
reddened skin, _____.
white blood cell, _____.
blue-bloodedness, _____.

91.

Now try these qualifiers.

hypertrophia	atrophy
general	systemic
local	

general or systemic
hypertrophia

local

systemic

atrophy

pertaining to the entire body _____.
overdevelopment _____.
pertaining to a small area, or one part,

_____.

pertaining to all body systems

_____.

a wasting away, underdevelopment,

_____.

92.

Here are some strictly objective symptoms.

tinnitus   malaise
emesis   nausea
vertigo   anorexia

vertigo

a sensation of turning around in space
_____.

nausea

seasickness; inclined to vomit
_____.

emesis

another word for vomitus _____.

tinnitus

ringing in the ears _____.

malaise

a vague sensation of not feeling well
_____.

anorexia

loss of appetite _____.

93.

A diagnosis is an identification of an illness. It requires scientific and skillful methods to establish the cause and nature of a sick person's disease. A diagnosis is arrived at by evaluating (a) the history of the person's disease, (b) the signs and symptoms present, (c) laboratory data, and (d) special tests such as X rays and electrocardiograms.

94.

In your English dictionary, you'll find words beginning with gnos. They come from the Greek word *gnosis* meaning knowledge. Dia means through. Therefore, dia/gnosis literally means

knowing through

_____.

95.

Diagnosing an illness means studying it through its signs and symptoms and other available information. When a patient reports chills, feels hot, and has a runny nose, the physician may identify the patient's illness as a head cold. This conclusion would be the _____.

diagnosis
dī ag nō´ sis

96.

A patient complains of pain in her arm after falling off her horse. An X ray shows a broken bone in her forearm. With this information from an X ray, the physician arrives at a _____.

diagnosis

identification of a
  patient's illness
  through blood
  (studies)

97.

What do you think hemodiagnosis means?

_____

_____.

98.

Many diseases are complex, so establishing the cause and nature of a sick person's disease requires skill and scientific methods. Which of the following might a physician use to help identify an illness? Check one or more.

all are relevant

_____ personal and family history
_____ signs and symptoms
_____ laboratory data
_____ special tests, such as an X ray or ECG

one who is skilled
  in making
  diagnoses

99.

If an obste/trician is one who is skilled in delivering babies, what is a dia/gnos/tician?

_____.

(Here's our
   suggestion)
to predict the
   patient's illness
   (its course and
   outcome)

100.
The prefix pro- means before, or in front of. What
do you think is the meaning of pro/gnosis?

_____

_____.

prognosis
prog nō´ sis

101.
Acute leukemia is often fatal within three months.
Prediction of the course and outcome of this
disease is called a _____.

to tell what the
   course and likely
   outcome of the
   disease will be

102.
What does prognosticate mean? _____

_____

_____.

103.
A prognosis predicts the course and outcome of a
disease. Select a term that best fits each outcome
described.

   favorable   unfavorable   guarded

Expect the patient to die in 3 to 6 months

unfavorable   _____.

Recovery will be easy after surgery

favorable   _____.

Recovery will be long and difficult

guarded   _____.

104.
A patient who has little chance of recovering from
his disease is said to have an (two words)

unfavorable
   prognosis

_____ _____.

105.
When a physician has identified the patient's illness, the physician has made a

diagnosis

_____.

106.
Prediction of the course and outcome of the disease

prognosis

is a _____.

107.
A diagnosis may specify that the disease is acute, chronic, or paroxysmal.

Acute means sharp, severe, having a rapid onset and a short course, not chronic.

Chronic means long, drawn out. A chronic disease is not acute.

Paroxysmal is from the Greek word *paroxysm*. It means a sudden periodic attack or recurrence of symptoms of disease; a fit or convulsion of any kind.

108.
Diabetes is a disease that has a long, drawn-out course. Therefore, diabetes is a

chronic
kron´ ik

_____ disease.
(acute / chronic / paroxysmal)

109.
Epilepsy is characterized by a sudden onset of symptoms that recur periodically. Therefore,

paroxysmal
par ok sis´ mal

epilepsy is a _____ illness.
(acute / chronic / paroxysmal)

110.

suddenly recurring episode of difficult breathing

Dys/pnea means difficult breathing. Paroxysmal dyspnea is another way to describe asthma. Explain paroxysmal dyspnea. _____

_____

_____.

111.

stomach

Gastritis may be acute or chronic. Acute gastritis means inflammation of the _____.

rapid

Its onset is _____, the pain in the
(rapid / slow)

severe

belly is _____, and the illness
(mild / severe)

short

lasts a _____ time.
(short / long)

112.

paroxysmal tachy/cardia

A patient has a sudden onset of fast heart rate—in excess of 200 beats per minute—and then abruptly the heart rate returns to normal. This has occurred before. The diagnosis would be

_____ _____ / _____.

(acute / chronic / paroxysmal)   rapid   heart

113.

chronic

Arteriosclerotic heart disease (ASHD) has a very slow onset. Symptoms may be mild and last a lifetime. ASHD is a /an _____ condition.

114.

Inflammatory conditions may be either acute or chronic. Acute tendonitis means the tendon becomes red, hot, and very painful in a few hours. It returns to normal after a day or two of treatment.

inflammation that
  has a slow onset
  (may be mild)
  and lasts a long
  time

Describe chronic tendonitis: _____

_____

_____.

---

paroxysm
par´ ok sizm

115.

A fit or convulsion is a/an _____.
A long, drawn-out disease is described as

chronic

_____.

Sharp, severe symptoms, over a short course,

acute

describes a/an _____ disease.

116.

Poly- is a prefix meaning many or much; excessive. Explain each of the following:

an inflammation of
  many nerves, a
  rapid onset; very
  painful, short
  duration

Acute polyneuritis means _____

_____

_____.

an inflammation of
  many joints that
  starts slowly and
  lasts a long time

Chronic polyarthritis _____

_____

_____.

a condition of
  having
  supernumerary
  fingers (or toes)

Polydactylism _____

_____

_____.

117.

Syndrome is a group of symptoms that occur together and thus characterize a specific disease. Syn means together; drome means running along.

symptoms running
  along together

Therefore, syndrome literally means _____

_____.

118.
For example, Korsakoff's syndrome is a psychosis, ordinarily due to chronic alcoholism. It is characterized by polyneuritis, disorientation, insomnia, muttering delirium, hallucinations, and a bilateral wrist or foot drop. Korsakoff's syndrome is characterized by this group of symptoms that

together   occur _____.

119.
A syndrome is a variety of symptoms occurring together. When symptoms run along together, they present a complete picture of the disease. This is

syndrome   known as a _____.
sin´ drōm

120.
Alcoholism produces a characteristic group of symptoms called Korsakoff's syndrome. From the

symptoms   name we know that a variety of _____
together   occur _____.

121.
A group of symptoms occurring together characterize a specific disease. We call this group

syndrome   of symptoms a _____.

122.
Recurrent (and usually progressive) hearing loss, tinnitus, vertigo, and a sensation of fullness in the

syndrome   ears is known as Ménière's _____.
the symptoms run   Explain why: _____
   along together   _____.

123.
Pro/drome means running before (a disease). A symptom or group of symptoms may occur a few hours or a few days before the onset of the disease.

prodrome   These early signals are called its
prō´ drom   _____.

124.
The prodromal phase of a disease is the interval between the earliest symptoms and the appearance of a rash or fever. These symptoms occur

before
_____ the onset of the disease.
(before / after)

125.
prodrome
Sneezing that comes before the chills and fever of a common cold is the _____ of the cold.

126.

prodrom (al)
prō drō´ mal
Malaise, anorexia, and sore throat occur one to four days before the fever and rash of measles appear. This early stage of the disease is called the
_____al phase.

127.
It's time to review what you just covered. From the suggested answers, select the best term for each brief definition.

asymptomatic   acute
prognosis   prodromal
chronic   diagnose
syndrome   paroxysm

diagnose
paroxysm

to identify an illness, _____.
a sudden, recurrent attack, _____.
pertaining to severe symptoms and rapid onset,

acute
_____.

prognosis
prediction of course and outcome of illness,
_____.

symptoms occurring together as a disease,

syndrome
asymptomatic
_____.

relating to symptom free, _____.
pertaining to a long, drawn-out illness,

chronic
_____.

phase between earliest symptoms and fever or rash,

prodromal
_____.

128.
Using scientific and skillful methods of investigation, a physician gathers information about a patient's illness in order to learn the cause and nature of a sick person's disease. Identification
diagnosis   of the illness is called a _____ .

Treatment

Treatment is the medical, surgical, or psychiatric management of a patient's illness. Although there are many different kinds of treatments, we're covering only a few of the most common.

129.
Active treatment aims for a cure. A patient suffering from appendicitis expects to be cured after an appendectomy. Since surgery removes the patient's appendix and usually cures the patient's
active   disease, it is an _____ treatment.

130.
An antibiotic attacks the bacteria causing peritonitis. Therefore, antibiotic therapy is
active   considered an _____ treatment.

131.
Systemic treatment attacks constitutional signs and symptoms such as pyrexia, shock, and pain.
systemic   Treatment directed toward control of these life-
sis tem´ ik   threatening signs is called _____ treatment.

132.
Giving a patient morphine for pain is a systemic treatment that aims to relieve a

life-threatening or
constitutional

_____ sign or symptom.

133.
Hyperpyrexia is a constitutional sign. Placing a hyperpyrexic child in a basin of ice water reduces the whole body temperature and is therefore a

systemic

_____ treatment.

134.
Palliative treatment relieves bothersome symptoms and makes a patient comfortable. Very little the physician can do alters the course of poison ivy dermatitis. The physician may suggest calamine

palliative
pal´ ē a tiv

lotion to reduce itching and burning, and therefore, calamine is called a _____ treatment.

135.
Prophylaxis is a treatment modality that focuses on prevention of disease. Your dentist aims to prevent dental caries by applying flouride solution to your

prophylactic
prō fi lak´ tic

teeth. Flouride application is called a _____ treatment.

136.
Whether active, symptomatic, palliative, or prophylactic, things the physician does or prescribes to manage a patient's illness are called

treatments

_____.

137.
Palliative treatment addresses a patient's comfort rather than attempting to cure the disease. The purpose of this kind of treatment is to

relieve symptoms

_____.

138.
Active treatment squarely addresses the patient's
pathological condition. The physician elects an
active treatment modality when a remedy or
therapy will _____ the disease.

cure
kyo͞or

139.
Shock, pyrexia, and pain are indications of disease,
which if not treated could have very serious
consequences. Systemic treatment is directed
toward very serious constitutional signs of illness

life-threatening
which may be _____.

140.
From the terms listed, select one that best fits each
description.

active   palliative
prophylactic   systemic

Treatment of constitutional symptoms,

systemic
_____.

Treatment directed specifically toward a cure,

active
_____.

Treatment to relieve discomfort,

palliative
_____.

Treatment aimed at preventing disease,

prophylactic
_____.

141.
There are many remedies and therapies a physician
may use to treat a patient's illness. Here are a few
of the major classes for you to investigate. Look up
therapy in your medical dictionary.

pharmcotherapy   radiotherapy
physical therapy   electroshock therapy
chemotherapy   psychotherapy

Statistics

In medicine and health care, many people keep score. The Health and Human Services Agency (HHS) of the U.S. government and the World Health Organization (WHO) of the United Nations publish statistics showing how many people are affected by certain diseases and how many people die of their illnesses. In order to understand the statistics, there are two important terms to know: morbidity and mortality.

morbidity (or
sickness)
mor bid´ i tē

142.
Morbidity means a diseased state. A statistic that reports, "50 cases of measles per 10,000 people living in the United States last year" is called a
_____ rate.

mortality (or death)
mor tal´ i tē

143.
Mortality means the state of being mortal and, therefore, subject to death. In other words, mortality is a statistic that reports the _____ rate.

all three are
mortality
statistics

144.
Which of the following examples expresses a mortality rate? Check each correct example.

a. _____ From 198X to 199X, 3 million people were killed in automobile accidents on U.S. highways.

b. _____ Hepatitis took the lives of 20 people of every 1,000 in Ethiopia in 198X.

c. _____ Thirty thousand children around the world died of leukemia in the last five years.

death

145.
The mortality rate is the same as saying the
_____ rate.

sickness or disease

146.
The morbidity rate is expressed as the number of
cases of a specific disease found in a specific unit
of population during a specific period of time. It
shows the rate of _____.

a. reports rate of
sickness

147.
Which of the following examples is a morbidity
rate? Check each correct example.

a. _____ In 198X, there were 550 new cases of
tuberculosis reported for every 100,000 people
living in the United States.

b. _____ In 198X, there were 30 deaths from
suicide for every 10,000 people between 35 and 55
years of age living in Colorado.

morbidity
rate

148.
A statistic that reports the number of cases of a
disease in a specific population for a specific
period of time is called _____
_____.

mortality rate

149.
A statistic that reports the death rate is called
_____ _____.

morbidity refers to
the rate of
illness;
mortality refers to
the death rate

150.
What is the difference between a morbidity and a
mortality statistic? _____
_____
_____.

151.

In this unit you worked with many new terms and learned to use some familiar words in new ways. Fifty of these words are listed here for you to practice your pronunciation and to review their meanings. Pronounce each term, think about its meaning, and then take the Unit 6 Self-Test.

acute (a kūt´)
anorexia (an o rek´ sē ə)
antipyretic (an tē pī ret´ ik)
asymptomatic (ā simp tō mat´ ik)
atrophy (at´ rō fē)
bradypnea (brad´ ip nē ə)
central (sen´ trul)
Cheyne-Stokes respiration
    (chān-stōks)
chlorocyte (klor´ ō sīt)
chronic (kron´ ik)
cyanoderma (sī ə nō der´ mä)
diagnosis (dī ag nō´ sis)
dyspnea (disp´ nē ə)
edema (e dē´ mä)
emesis (em´ ə sis)
erythremia (er i thrē´ mē ə)
generalized
hyperpnea (h perp´ nē ə)
hyperpyrexia (hī per pī rek´ sē ə)
hypothermia (hī pō ther´ mē ə)
leukocyte (loo´ kō sīt)
localized
malaise (mä lāz´)
melanocarcinoma
    (mel´ ə nō kär sin ō´ mä)

morbidity (mor bid´ i tē)
mortality (mor tal´ i tē)
nausea (naw´ zē ə)
palliative (pal´ ē ə tiv)
paroxysmal (par ok sis´ mal)
peripheral (per i´ fer al)
pneometer (nē om´ ə ter)
polyarthritis (pol´ ē arth rī´ tis)
prodromal (prō drō´ mal)
prognosis (prog nō´ sis)
prophylactic (prō fi lak´ tic)
pulse (pultz´)
pyretic (pī ret´ ik)
pyretolysis (pī ret ō lī´ sis)
pyrexia (pī rek´ sē ə)
respiration
symptom
symptomatic
syndrome (sin´ drōm)
systemic
tachypnea (tak ip nē´ ə)
temperature
tinnitus (ti nī´ tus)
vertigo (ver´ ti gō)
vital signs
xanthopsia (zan thop´ sē ə)

Unit 6: Self-Test

PART 1

From the list on the right, select the correct meaning for each of the
following medical terms.

_____   1. Diagnosis
_____   2. Systemic
_____   3. Morbidity
_____   4. Pyretolysis
_____   5. Edema
_____   6. Generalized
_____   7. Anorexia
_____   8. Vertigo
_____   9. Hyperpnea
_____ 10. Malaise
_____ 11. Cyanoderma
_____ 12. Vital signs
_____ 13. Syndrome
_____ 14. Nausea
_____ 15. Atrophy

a. Bluish color of skin
b. Pertaining to the whole body,
   all systems
c. Ringing in the ear
d. Identification of an illness
e. Fluid in the tissues
f. Pertaining to disease rate
   statistic
g. Temperature, pulse, and
   respiration
h. Reduction of fever
i. A sickness of the stomach;
   desire to vomit
j. Excessively fast breathing
k. Pertaining to the whole body,
   many different parts at the
   same time
l. Wasting away, or
   underdevelopment
m. Loss of appetite
n. Sensation of turning around in
   space
o. Vague sensation of not feeling
   well
p. Pertaining to sudden periodic
   attack
q. Symptoms occurring together

PART 2

Complete each of the medical terms on the right with the appropriate
missing part. Some terms are missing all parts!

1. Ringing in the ear   _____
2. Artery throbbing in time with
   the heartbeat   _____
3. Respiratory arrest, not breathing   _____
4. Outside surface of the body   _____
5. Pertaining to preventing disease   _____
6. Sudden recurring attack   P_____
7. Symptom free   _____
8. Breathing that reaches a
   climax, then ceases before   C_____-S_____
   beginning again   respiration
9. Pertaining to relieving symptoms
   but not the disease   _____
10. Perceived change in body or
    functions   _____
11. Prediction of course and
    outcome of a disease   _____
12. Pertaining to severe symptoms,
    rapid onset, short course   _____
13. Reddened skin   E_____
14. Subnormal body temperature
    under 90°F   _____
15. Feverishness   _____

ANSWERS

Part 1

1. d
2. b
3. f
4. h
5. e
6. k
7. m
8. n

9. j
10. o
11. a
12. g
13. q
14. i
15. l

Part 2

1. Tinnitus
2. Pulse
3. Apnea
4. Peripheral
5. Prophylactic
6. Paroxysm
7. Asymptomatic
8. Cheyne-Stokes respiration

9. Palliative
10. Symptom
11. Prognosis
12. Acute
13. Erythroderma
14. Hypothermia
15. Pyrexia

Unit 7

In this unit you will learn terms relating to growth and development and other kinds of growing things. Then you'll cover terms which provide an orientation to the body in the same way that points on the compass make a road map meaningful.

ecto- (*outer side*)
endo- (*inner side*)
meso- (*middle*)

circum- (*around*)
peri- (*around about*)

epi- (*over, surrounding*)
sub-, hypo- (*below, under*)
supra-, super- (*above, over*)
infra- (*below, beneath*)

Growth and Development

1.
Blastos means a germ or a seed. A blastoderm is an aggregation of cells showing the first trace of organization. It is the most rudimentary form of a developing embryo and is made up of three primary germ layers: the ectoderm, endoderm, and mesoderm. It is from these primordial germ layers that the embryo becomes a fetus.

2.
Review the table and then complete frames 3 to 13. Refer back to the table for help as you need it.

DEVELOPMENT OF FETAL TISSUE

ECTODERM
1. Epidermis
2. Epithelium of:
   external and internal ear
   nasal cavity
   mouth
   anus
   amnion, chorion
   distal part of male urethra
3. Nervous tissue

MESODERM
1. Connective tissues
2. Male and female reproductive tracts
3. Blood vessels, lymphatics
4. Kidneys, ureters, trigone of bladder
5. Pleura, peritoneum, pericardium
6. Muscles

ENDODERM (ENTODERM)
1. Respiratory tract except nose
2. Digestive tract except mouth and anus
3. Bladder except trigone
4. Male urethra, proximal portion
5. Female urethra

3.

Ectoderm is the outer layer of cells. Endoderm is the innermost of the three germ layers. Mesoderm is the middle layer of three primary germ layers in the developing embryo. Write a meaning for each of the prefixes:

inner, inside	endo- means _____.
middle	meso- means _____.
outside	ecto- means _____.

4.

Which primary germ layer originates all connective tissues and all body musculature?

mesoderm
mēz´ ō derm

_____.

5.
The pleura is a watery, mucoid-surfaced membrane enveloping the lungs and lining the walls of the pleural cavity. From which germ layer does it arise? _____.

mesoderm

6.
Which of the three embryonic germ layers gives rise to the nervous system and the organs of special sense? _____.

ectoderm
ek′ tō derm

7.
The primative gut tract and its associated glands (organs) develop from which germ layer of the embryo? _____.

endoderm
en′ dō derm

8.
The skin, including mucous membranes exposed to the environment, are derived from the primary germ layer called the _____.

ectoderm

9.
The innermost of the three primary germ layers of the embryo is the _____. The outside layer of cells in the embryo is the _____. The middle of the three primary germ layers is the _____.

endoderm

ectoderm
mesoderm
mēz′ ō derm

10.
Now let's try out those new prefixes. Write a meaning for each of the following:
ectocytic _____
_____.

outside the cell
inflammation of
   inside of the
   heart

endocarditis _____
_____.

examination by
   looking inside of
   (a body cavity)

endoscopy _____
_____.

examination of
   inside the
   bladder

endocystoscopy _____
_____.

11.

Gen/o is the word root meaning to originate.

originating outside
of
ek toj´ en us

Ectogenous means _____

_____.

originating from
inside of
en doj´ en us

Endogenous means _____

_____.

12.

Topos, top/o means place or location. Sometimes a pregnancy begins in the fallopian tube instead of within the uterus. It is called an ectopic pregnancy.

pregnancy out of
its normal
location

What is an ectopic pregnancy? _____

_____.

13.

A pregnancy beginning in the abdominal cavity instead of the womb is called an

ectopic
ek top´ ik

_____ pregnancy.

14.

Let's review before going on. From the suggested answers, select the best term for each brief definition.

SUGGESTED ANSWERS:

ecto-	endo-
ectopic	endocranial
ectocytic	endogenous
meso-	mesoderm

ecto-
meso-
endo-
mesoderm
endogenous
ectocytic
ectopic
endocranial

outside (prefix), _____.
middle (prefix), _____.
inside (prefix), _____.
middle germ cell layer, _____.
originating inside, _____.
pertaining to outside the cell, _____.
out of its normal place, _____.
pertaining to inside the head, _____.

Growths and Other Abnormal Tissues

15.
In this section you'll work with more terms relating to growth. Growing means to increase progressively in size. However, growth may be normal and purposeful, or abnormal and useless. Here are some terms used to describe abnormal growth.

16.
Neo- means new; -plasm means thing formed. Neoplasm is a new formation of tissue. It is abnormal because it serves no useful function and grows at the expense of a healthy body. Any tissue growing autonomously and that has no useful function is a _____.

neoplasm
nē´ ō plazm

17.
A tumor is a swelling or enlargement. It is an autonomous new growth of tissue. It is a mass of tissue without a function. Another word for tumor is _____.

neoplasm

18.
Neoplasm and tumor are interchangeable terms. They both mean an autonomous new _____ _____.

growth of tissue
    that serves no
    useful purpose

19.
Bio- means life; -opsy means appearance, sight. A biopsy is removing tissue from a living body and examining it under a microscope.

To make a diagnosis, a physician usually biopsies a tumor or neoplasm. This means the physician removes a piece of living _____ and _____ it under a microscope.

tissue
examines

20.

A neoplasm (tumor) growing in or on the human body can be classified as either malignant or benign.

Malignant means it's of a bad kind, growing worse, resisting treatment, and tending or threatening to produce death.

benign
bē nīn´
malignant
ma lig´ nant

Benign means it's mild (grows slowly), not spreading, not recurrent, and not malignant. Tumors may be of uncertain behavior, but usually are classified either as _____ or

_____ .

21.

To determine what kind of neoplasm a patient has, the physician removes a piece of the living tumor tissue and examines it under a microscope. What is

biopsy

this procedure called? _____ .

22.

A biopsy report indicates a patient's abnormal growth is of a bad kind. It will grow worse (rapidly), resist treatment, and tend to be life threatening. The diagnosis is

malignant

_____ neoplasm.

(malignant / benign)

23.

A nonmalignant neoplasm is an abnormal tissue mass growing slowly, not spreading, and not likely

benign

to recur. The growth is _____ .

(malignant / benign)

24.

A procedure that determines whether a neoplasm

biopsy

is benign or malignant is a _____ .

25.

fast

A malignant neoplasm is a bad kind that grows

_____, resists treatment, and

(fast / slowly)

death

threatens to cause _____.

26.

A benign neoplasm is mild (grows slowly), does
not spread or recur, and is not

malignant

_____.

(the other kind)

27.

Infiltration means slipping into and between
normal cells of the body.

Malignant tumor cells spread by slipping into and
between normal body cells. Malignant cells
multiply rapidly, take up nourishment and space,
crowding out the normal cells. This method of
spreading is called direct extension or

infiltration

_____.

28.

Meta- means after, beyond, among, over; -stasis
means a standing, a location, or place.

Metastasis means movement of cells (especially
cancer cells) from one part of the body to another.
Malignant tumor cells migrate to another location
and take up a standing in another organ or part of

metastasis

the body. This method of spreading the disease is

me tas´ tə sis

called invasion by _____.

29.

Metastasis is the movement of malignant tumor
cells from the primary location over to another

location

_____.

30.
There are two methods by which a malignant neoplasm spreads, grows larger, and becomes more threatening. Malignant cells may slip into and between normal cells. This is called _____. Or tumor cells may move beyond the primary site and take up a standing in another location of the body. This spreading method is called _____.

infiltration or
   direct extension

metastasis

31.
Unlike malignant neoplasms, benign growths do not spread by _____ or _____.

infiltration
metastasis

32.
Here's a quick review. Select a term from the suggested answers that best fits each brief definition. Write your selection in the space provided.

malignant	neoplasm/tumor
tumor/neoplasm	biopsy
benign	infiltration
metastasize	

remove tissue for examination,
_____.

biopsy

slow growth, not malignant,
_____.

benign

new, abnormal tissue mass,
_____.

neoplasm/tumor

tissue mass, no useful purpose,
_____.

tumor/neoplasm

fast growing, threatening death,
_____.

malignant

slipping into and between normal cells,
_____.

infiltration
metastasize
(me tās´ tə sīz)

cells relocate to new location, organ,
_____.

33.
There are many other terms that mean abnormal conditions, changes, or growths. Here are a few of the more common ones.

34.
Lesion is an area of unhealthy (morbid) tissue, such as an injury, wound, burn, or infected patch of skin.

Any morbid change in the structure of an organ or a part due to injury or disease is called a

lesion
lē´ zhun
_____.

35.
An infected finger is a lesion because there has been a morbid change in the finger tissues. What does morbid mean? _____.

diseased,
   unhealthy

36.
In Alzheimer's disease there are morbid changes in brain tissue. These unhealthy changes in brain structure are also called _____.

lesions

37.
An injury, a burn, and an infected finger are examples of lesions because the part of the body involved has undergone a _____
change.   (unhealthy)

morbid

38.
A lesion is any morbid change in the structure of an organ or part due to injury or disease. Check each item that is *not* a lesion.

ⓧ chicken pox is a
   disease; the pox
   are lesions

- ☐ duodenal ulcer
- ☐ skinned knees
- ☐ scalding burn of the hand
- ☐ abrasion of the elbow
- ☐ chicken pox
- ☐ infected toenail

39.
Poison ivy leaves irritate the skin and cause
unhealthy changes. These changes in the structure
lesions   of the skin are called _____.

40.
Build a word meaning a hurt, an injury, or any
unhealthy area of any organ or part:
lesion   _____.

unhealthy,   **41.**
   diseased   What does morbid mean? _____.

42.
In earlier units you learned that cyst means
bladder.
inflammation of   Cystitis means _____
   the bladder   _____.
examination of the   Endocystoscopy means _____
   inside of the   _____
   bladder   _____.
excision (or   Cholecystectomy means _____
   removal) of the   _____
   gallbladder   _____.

43.
Cyst also means a closed sac or pouch that contains
fluid, semifluid, or solid material. Cyst refers to an
abnormal development of a structure, obstruction
of ducts, and sometimes infections.
sac   A cyst is a closed _____.
fluid, semifluid, or It contains _____
   solid material   _____
                     _____.

Cyst

44.

A malfunctioning ovary may form a closed sac or pouch containing fluid. This is called an ovarian

cyst   _____.

45.

a cyst containing   What is a hydrocyst? _____
    fluid (water)

a sac that contains   _____.
    fluid or even   Cyst means _____
    solid material
                                _____.

46.

A physician doesn't usually drain a cyst of its contents because it only would fill again. Instead, a surgeon completely excises the cyst. Write a term meaning surgical removal of a cyst:

cystectomy   _____.

47.

pol´ip   Polyp is a tumor with a little foot, or stem. A polyp is usually a benign tumor. That means it is not

malignant   _____,
                             (the other kind)

                  it grows

slowly   _____,
                         (fast / slowly)

                  and it does *not* spread by
infiltration   _____ or
metastasis   _____.

Polyp

48.

A polyp is a specific type of tumor or neoplasm. It's an abnormal, useless new growth that stands on a
foot   stem or a little _____.

49.
Vascular organs such as the nose, uterus, and rectum commonly develop polyps. Polyps bleed easily and usually are removed surgically. Build a word for excision of polyps:

polypectomy

_____.

50.

unhealthy

A lesion is an area of _____ tissue.

burn, injury,
   infection

Give some examples of lesions: _____

_____.

51.
Cyst has two different meanings.

bladder

Cyst means _____.
                          a part of the body

a sac containing
   fluid or
   semifluid

Cyst also means

_____.
                          an abnormality

52.

tumor/neoplasm
little foot

A polyp is a specific kind of _____.
A polyp has a _____.

53.
Papilla is a small nipplelike protuberance or elevation. It may be located anywhere on the body, and may be normal or abnormal.

Papilla

Taste buds are small nipplelike structures on the surface of the tongue. They account for the four fundamental taste sensations: sweet, bitter, sour, and salt. Stand in front of a mirror; stick your tongue way out. You will see papillae (plural) on the back of your tongue. Describe them:

small, nipplelike structures

_____.

54.
The nipple of the mammary gland (breast) is called a mammary _____.

papilla
pa pil´ ə

55.
Papilloma is a hypertrophied papilla covered by a layer of skin. What is the shape of a papilloma?

_____.

pap i lō´ mä

nipplelike

56.
Papule is a pimple. It's a red elevated spot on the skin. It's solid and circumscribed. Papular lesions appear on the skin in smallpox, measles, and chicken pox.

pap´ yo͞ol

Papule

They are elevated red _____.

spots
circumscribed

They are solid and _____.

57.

Excrescence: ex means out; crescence means to grow. Excrescence is a useless structure growing out of the surface of a part such as a wart or mole.

The Wicked Witch of the West had a big wart growing on the tip of her nose. A medical term for this disfiguring outgrowth is

excrescence
eks kres´ ens

_____.

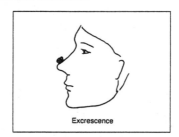

Excrescence

58.

Condyloma is a wartlike growth of the skin, usually occurring near the anus. The main difference between an excrescence and a condyloma is where the lesion is located. An excrescence may appear anywhere on the surface of the body (even on the end of your nose). But a wartlike skin growth near the anus is called a _____.

kon di lō´ mä
condyloma

59.

An excrescence, a papilloma, a condyloma, and a papule are all lesions of the skin. That means the area of the skin involved is considered

morbid, unhealthy

_____.

60.

pa pil´ ē (pl.)

Papillae (plural) may be normal structures on the body that have important functions. A taste bud is a papilla. Describe what it looks like:

small, nipplelike
    protuberance

_____.

(For help in learning the plural forms, see Appendix B: _Forming Plurals._)

61.
Label each of the following illustrations.

a. cyst
b. polyp

a. _____   b. _____

c. papilla
d. papule

c. _____   d. _____

62.
Complete each definition.

SUGGESTED ANSWERS

papillae	condyloma
excrescence	lesion
polyp	papule
cyst	

lesion (lē´ zhun)

area of unhealthy (morbid) tissue,
_____.

polyp (pol´ ip)
condyloma
   (kon di lō´ mä)

tumor on a stem or little foot,
_____.

wartlike growth around the anus,
_____.

cyst (sist)
excrescence
   (eks kres´ ens)

bladder, or a closed sac with fluid,
_____.

useless outgrowth, like a wart,
_____.

papillae (pa pil´ ē)

nipplelike protuberances,
_____.

papule (pap´ yōōl)

small, elevated red lesion on the skin,
_____.

63.

Here's an independent learning exercise for you.
These are words related to treatments and
consequences of malignant neoplasms. Look up
each one in your medical dictionary. Explore it
thoroughly; pronounce it several times. Then write
a brief definition for each. Do this exercise even if
you think you know what the terms mean.
Sometimes you'll be surprised!

abdominal paracentesis

_____
_____.

alopecia

_____
_____.

anastomosis

_____
_____.

cauterization

_____
_____.

chemotherapy

_____
_____.

dehiscence

_____
_____.

necrobiosis

_____
_____.

radiation

_____
_____.

radical resection

_____
_____.

Orientation

64.
Neoplasms, cysts, and lesions occur anywhere on the surface of the body and inside, under, and around organs and structures. Physicians use specific terms to describe where parts of the body are located relative to other parts of the body.

65.
Ventral means on or near the belly, or the side of the body where the belly is located.

back

Dorsal is the opposite of ventral; it means on or near the _____.

Label the illustrations.

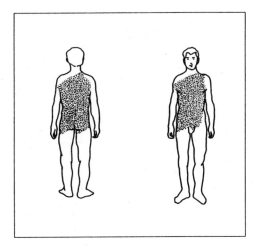

a. dorsal
b. ven´tral
    ven´tral

a. _____   b. _____

belly
back

66.
Ventral, ventr/o means on or near the _____. Dorsal, dors/o means on or near the _____.

67.
Try these.

backache
incision into the
   belly

Dorsalgia means _____.

Ventrotomy means _____

_____.

68.
What do you think ventrodorsad means?

belly to back

_____.

A bullet penetrated the abdominal wall, traveled
through the belly, and exited through the back.

ventrodorsad
ven trō dor´ säd

The bullet's path may be called

_____.

69.
The midline, or median, is an imaginary line
dividing the body into right
and left halves.

Lateral means farther from the
midline.

Medial means the opposite.

Medial means

nearer

_____ to the
midline.

Which is nearer the midline,
your shoulder or your nipple ?

nipple

_____.

70.
Which corner of your eye is nearest your ear?

lateral

_____.

Which side of your knee knocks the other knee?

medial

_____.

71.

farther

Lateral means _____ from the midline.

nearer

Medial means _____ to the midline.

Where is your umbilicus located?

on the midline

_____.

72.

Let's describe a relative position in another way.

Distal means remote, or farthest, from the point of attachment to the trunk.

Proximal means the opposite. Proximal means

nearest

_____ to the point of

(farthest / nearest)

attachment to the trunk.

73.

Which is distal, your elbow or your hand?

hand

_____.

On which end of your finger do you wear a ring?

proximal

_____.

74.

Your forearm bone has two ends. Your hand is

distal

attached to the _____ end.

(distal / proximal)

Your upper arm is located on the

proximal

_____ end.

(distal / proximal)

75.

A part of the body located nearest its attachment to

proximal

the trunk is described as _____.

A part located farthest from its attachment to the

distal

trunk is described as _____.

76.

farthest from the
attachment to
the trunk

The fingers are distal to all other parts of the arm.
What does distal mean? _____

_____.

77.

nearest to the
attachment to
the trunk

Describe the location of a part that is proximal:

_____

_____.

78.

Here's a review of what you just covered. Select the
best term from the suggested answers to complete
each definition.

SUGGESTED ANSWERS:

distal	proximal
medial	lateral
ventral	midline
dorsal	

dorsal
ventral

near, or on the back, _____.
near, or on the belly, _____.
divides body into right and left halves,

midline
lateral
medial

_____.
farther from the midline, _____.
nearer to the midline, _____.
farthest from the attachment to the trunk,

distal

_____.
nearest to the attachment to the trunk,

proximal

_____.

79.

Here are some prefixes indicating place or relative
position:
Peri-, circum- means around, about, surrounding,

Write a meaning for each of the following:

pertaining to
around the tonsil
relating to around
the belly button

Peri/tonsillar _____

_____.

Peri/umbilical _____

_____.

diseased
  (unhealthy)
  tissue around
  the teeth
around

80.
What is peri/dent/al (peri/dont/al) gum disease?

_____

_____.

Peri- means _____.

around

moving around

81.
Circum- is another prefix meaning

_____. Duct/ion means moving.

Ab/duct/ion is moving away. Circum/duction

means _____.

circum(-scribed)

82.
A wheal (hives) is a round patch of unhealthy skin
that becomes normal tissue at its circumference. A
wheal appears as a round red spot. We usually say
a wheal is _____-scribed.

circumscribed

83.
A boil also has an outer limit where the
circumference of the lesion becomes normal.
Because it appears to have a border around its
circumference, you may also describe a boil as a
_____ lesion.

relating to around
  the mouth
pertaining to
  around the
  kidney

84.
Perioral and circumoral have the same meaning.
Write the meaning: _____

_____.

Write a meaning for circumrenal, perirenal:

_____

_____.

85.
Look over the following terms and their meanings and then complete frames 86 to 94. Come back to this table whenever you need help.

Epi-	upon, over (surrounding or covering)
Extra-	without, outside of
Infra-	below, beneath, under
Sub-, hypo-	below, beneath, less than normal
Supra-, super-	above, superior, in the upper part of

86.
The epi/gastric region is the region of the belly over or upon the stomach. Refer to the illustration in frame 95.

pain in the area of
the belly over
the stomach

Epi/gastralgia means _____
_____
_____.

hernia in the area
of the belly over
the stomach

Epi/gastrocele means _____
_____
_____.

87.
Epi/cranium refers to the tissues (muscle and skin) that cover and surround the cranium. What do you think epi/dermis means? _____

the skin (that
covers the entire
body)

_____.

88.
Again refer to the definitions in frame 85.

without,
outside of

The prefix extra- means _____
_____.

outside the uterus

Extra/uterine means _____
_____.

outside the edges
or outer limits of
a structure or
organ

Extra/marginal means _____
_____
_____.

89.

below, beneath,
  under

Again use the definitions in frame 85 to help you.
The prefix infra- means _____.
Patella means kneecap. What does infra/patellar

under, below the
  kneecap

mean? _____
_____.

beneath, under the
  kneecap

Sub/patellar means _____
_____.

90.

Infra- and sub- usually are interchangeable terms.
Complete the alternate terms and write a meaning:

infra (-mammary)

_____-mammary

sub (-mammary)

_____- mammary

below the breast

meaning _____.

91.

Sub- and hypo- are often interchangeable also.
Sub/lingual means

under the tongue

_____.

Hypo/glossal means

under the tongue

_____.

92.

below, beneath,
  less than normal

The prefix sub- means _____
_____. What other two prefixes
often are interchangeable and mean the same thing

infra-,

as sub- ? _____ and

hypo-

_____.

93.

Sternum is the breastbone. Write a meaning for

pertaining to below
  the breastbone

sub/sternal: _____
_____.

Use another prefix and build another term that

infrasternal

means the same thing: _____.

94.

Build a term that means pertaining to above the sternum: _____.

suprasternal

Regions of the Abdomen

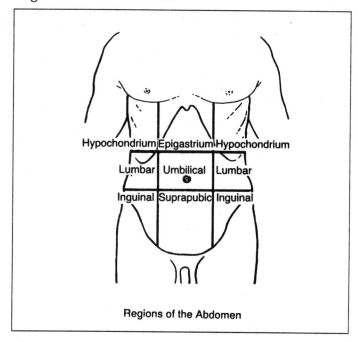

Regions of the Abdomen

95.

Refer to the illustration to help you complete frames 96 to 99.

96.

Sub/pubic refers to an area beneath the pubic arch (bone). Build a term meaning relating to the area above the pubic arch: _____.

Umbilical is the term meaning relating to the area that is near/around the _____.

suprapubic
umbilicus or belly
button

97.
Chondros means cartilage (of ribs). Literally,
hypochondrium means the area _____

beneath the ribs   _____ .

98.
Lumbar relates to the loins. It is the part of the back
and sides between the ribs and the pelvis. What

inguinal
ing´ giwi nal   area is below the lumbar region?

_____ .

99.
Write a meaning for each of the following terms.

pertaining to
    around the   Peri/umbilical, _____
    umbilicus   _____ .

relating to under   Sub/abdominal, _____
    the stomach   _____ .

relating to above   Supra/lumbar, _____
    the loin   _____ .

pertaining to below   Infra/pubic, _____
    the pubic arch   _____ .
pertaining to
    around the   Circum/intestinal, _____
    intestine   _____ .

pertaining to under   Hypo/dermic, _____
    the skin   _____ .
relating to outside
    the field   Extra/visual, _____
    of vision   _____ .

100.

In this unit you worked with 36 new medical terms. Practice pronouncing them. Then take the Unit 7 Self-Test.

benign

biopsy

circumocular

circumscribed

condyloma (kon di lō′ mä)

cyst (sist)

distal

dorsal

ectoderm (ek tō derm)

ectopic (ek top′ ik)

endogenous (en doj′ ə nus)

endocystoscopy
    (en dō sis tos′ ko pē)

epigastric (ep ē gas′ trik)

excrescence (eks kres′ ens)

extrasensory (eks tra sen′ sō rē)

hypodermic (hī pō derm′ ik)

infiltration

inframammary (in fra mam′ ə rē)

lateral

lesion

lumbar

malignant (ma lig′ nant)

medial

mesoderm (mēz′ ō derm)

metastasis (me tas′ ta sis)

neoplasm (nē ō plazm)

papilla (pa pil′ ə)

papilloma (pap i lō′ mä)

papules (pap′ yōōls)

periumbilical (per′ ē um bil′ i k'l)

polyp (pol′ ip)

proximal (prox′ si mal)

subpatellar (sub pa tel′ ar)

suprapubic (su pra pyōō′ bik)

tumor

ventral

Unit 7 Self-Test

PART 1

From the right, select the correct meaning for each of the following often used medical terms.

_____ 1. Endocystoscopy
_____ 2. Lesion
_____ 3. Circumocular
_____ 4. Distal
_____ 5. Endocranial
_____ 6. Epigastric
_____ 7. Biopsy
_____ 8. Neoplasm
_____ 9. Ectoderm
_____ 10. Metastasis
_____ 11. Malignant
_____ 12. Benign
_____ 13. Infiltration
_____ 14. Proximal
_____ 15. Ectopic

a. Farthest point from trunk attachment
b. Outside layer of germ cells
c. Not spreading, not malignant
d. Pertaining to inside the head vault
e. Pertaining to around the eye
f. Slipping into and between normal cells
g. Pertaining to the area over the stomach
h. Cells spread to new location, organ
i. Removal of tissue for examination
j. New, abnormal tissue formation
k. Morbid tissue
l. Nearest the attachment to the trunk
m. A bad kind, tending to threaten death
n. Occurring outside the normal place
o. Examination inside the bladder

PART 2

Write the medical term for each of the following brief definitions.

1. Nipplelike protuberance — Pap_____
2. New, abnormal tissue without a purpose — _____
3. Useless structure growing out of the skin — Ex_____
4. Spread of cells to new location, organ — Meta_____
5. Pertaining to on or near the back — D_____
6. Farthest point from trunk attachment — D_____
7. Closed sac or pouch containing fluid — _____
8. Removal of tissue for examination — _____
9. Wartlike growth around the anus — C_____
10. Slipping into and between normal cells — In_____
11. Not spreading, not malignant — _____
12. Below the mammary gland — _____
13. Tumor with a little foot — P_____
14. Nearest point of trunk attachment — P_____
15. Unhealthy, diseased area of tissue — L_____

ANSWERS

Part 1

1. o	9. b
2. k	10. h
3. e	11. m
4. a	12. c
5. d	13. f
6. g	14. l
7. i	15. n
8. j	

Part 2

1. Papilla	9. Condyloma
2. Neoplasm/tumor	10. Infiltration
3. Excrescence	11. Benign
4. Metastasis	12. Inframammary
5. Dorsal	13. Polyp
6. Distal	14. Proximal
7. Cyst	15. Lesion
8. Biopsy	

Unit 8

This unit covers medical terms used in gynecology and obstetrics. You'll be working with the following new words, word roots, and prefixes:

-ary (*of or pertaining to*)
-atrophy (*undernourished, wasting*)
-dynia (*pain, painful*)
-mania (*madness*)
-pathy (*disease*)
-phobia (*excessive fear*)

primi- (*first*)
secundi- (*second*)
nulli- (*none*)
multi- (*many*)

amni/o, amniot/o (*fetal sac*)
gravid/a (*with child*)
gyn/o, gynec/o (*woman*)
hyster/o (*uterus*)
mamm/o (*breast*)
mast/o (*breast*)
men/o (*menses, menstruation*)
metr/o (*uterus*)
para (*bear, bring forth*)

pre- (*before*)
post- (*after*)
oligo- (*little, small, scanty*)

climacteric
conception
embryo
episiotomy
fetus
gestation
involution
labor

menopause
ovum
parturition
perineum
peritoneum
placenta
pudenda
puerperium

Terms of Gynecology

1.
Gyn, gynec/o means woman. Gynecology is the study of the female reproductive organs and breasts. Simply put, it is the field of medicine dealing with diseases of whom?

women
_____.

gī´ nō plas tē or
jin´ ō plas tē
plastic surgery of
female repro-
ductive organs

2.
Gyn/o/pathic means pertaining to diseases of women. What do you think gyn/o/plasty means?
_____
_____.

3.
Mania means madness. Phobia means excessive fear. Gynecomania is an abnormal sex drive and desire in the male of the species. What do you

gī ne fo´ bē a
fear of women

think gyne/phobia means? _____
_____.

gynecologist
gī ne kol´ ō jist

4.
The physician who specializes in female disorders is called a _____.

5.
Human beings are mammals. Mammals have glands that secrete milk for nourishing their offspring. In plain English, mammary gland means

breast
_____.

6.

These next two terms often are interchangeable. However, we use one term more often than the other. In this lesson you'll be using the preferred terms. Let's see what this means:

Mamm, mamm/o refers to mammary gland, or breast; mast, mast/o also refers to

breast   _____.

mam ī´ tis,
   mast ī´ tis
inflammation of
   the mammary
   gland (breast)
preferred

7.

Mamm/itis and mast/itis both mean

_____

_____.

Mastitis is the term used most often, so we say it is

the _____ term.

8.

Break down each of the following preferred terms and write its meaning.

ma mog´ ra fē
mamm/o/graphy
X ray exam of the
   breast
mas tek´ tō mē
mast/ectomy
surgical removal of
   a breast

Mammography, _____ / ___ / _____

means _____

_____

Mastectomy, _____ / _____

means _____

_____.

9.
Using the word roots mast, mast/o, add a suffix from the list and build a preferred term. Write its meaning in the space provided.

-otomy   -itis   -pathy

mastotomy
mas tot´ ō mē
incision into the
  breast

M _____

means _____

_____ ;

mastitis
inflammation of
  the breast

m _____

means _____

_____ ;

mastopathy
mas top´ a thē
disease of the
  mammary gland

m _____

means _____

_____ .

10.
Very large breasts that hang down, or droop, are described as pendulous. The suffix for hanging or drooping is -ptosis. Construct a word meaning

mastoptosis
mas top tō´ sis

pendulous breast: _____ .

11.
Here's an interesting term that doesn't follow the rules. Let's look at the parts. Gynec/o means woman; mastia means breast.

gī ne kō mas´ tē a
woman's breast

Gynecomastia literally means _____

_____ .

(In actual use it means abnormally large mammary glands in the male; sometimes they secrete milk.)

12.
This time use the word roots mamm, mamm/o.
Build a term with each of the following suffixes
and write its meaning:

          -gram   -ary

mam´ ō gram
    mammogram   M _____
X ray picture of the   means _____
    breast   _____;
mam´ a rē
    mammary   m _____
pertaining to the   means _____
    mammary gland   _____.

13.

mam´ ō plas tē
plastic surgery of
    the mammary
    gland

Mamm/o/pexy means surgical correction (fixation)
of large hanging breasts. What does
mamm/o/plasty mean? _____
_____

14.

mast´ ad nī tis
mast´ ad nō´ ma
tumor of the
    mammary gland
mas tō kar cin ō´
  ma
cancerous tumor of
    the mammary
    gland

Mast/aden/itis means inflammation of the
mammary gland. Write a meaning for each of the
following:

mastadenoma _____
_____;

mastocarcinoma _____
_____.

15.

mas tong´ kus
(any) tumor of the
    breast

Oncology is the study or science dealing with the
physical, chemical, and biologic properties of
neoplasms including causation, pathogenesis, and
treatment. What does mastoncus mean?
_____.

16.
Mast/o/dynia means painful breast. Using another suffix you know, build another word that also means pain in the breast:

mast/algia
mast al´ jē ə

mast/_____.

17.
Here's a quick review. Select a term from the suggested answers that best fits each brief definition. Write your selection in the space provided.

mastectomy   mastopathy
mastoptosis   gynecomastia
mastoncus   mastopexy

mastopathy
mas top´ a thē

disease of the mammary glands,

_____.

women's breasts (on a man),

gynecomastia

_____.

surgical removal of the breast,

mastectomy

_____.

pendulous breasts,

mastoptosis

_____.

any tumor of the breast,

mastoncus
mastopexy
mas´ tō pex´ sē

_____.

surgical fixation of pendulous breasts,

_____.

18.
Now try these.

mammoplasty   mammary
mammology   mammalgia (mastodynia)
mammography   gynecophobia

mammography
mammalgia
   (mastodynia)
mammology
gynecophobia
mammary

X ray study of the breast,

_____.

painful breast _____.

science and study of the breast,

_____.

fear of women, _____.

pertaining to the breast,

_____.

surgical reconstruction of the breast,

mammoplasty

_____.

Mamma mē´ a, you're doing very well!

19.
Female Genitourinary System

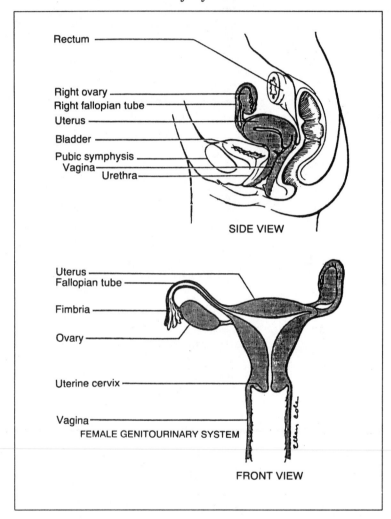

20.
Here are two more terms with nearly identical
meanings. Refer to the illustration in frame 19.

Hyster, hyster/o means uterus.
uterus   Metr, metr/o also means _____.

21.
Hyster/o usually refers to the uterus as a whole
organ. Metr/o usually refers to the tissues of the
uterus   _____.

22.
There are exceptions to the rule, but in general
whole   hyster/o means the uterus as a _____
tissues   organ. Metr/o refers to the _____
of the organ.

23.
Metr/itis means an inflammation of the uterine
tissues (linings, muscles, etc.). Metr/o/paralysis
(muscle) tissues of   means paralysis of _____
the uterus   _____.

24.
Hyster/o/tomy means incision into the uterus
(perhaps to remove a solid tumor). What does
muscle tumor of   hyster/o/my/oma mean? _____
the uterus   _____.

25.
Using the word roots hyster, hyster/o, add a suffix from the list and build a new word. Write its meaning in the space provided:

-ectomy   -pathy

hysterectomy
his ter rek´ tō mē   H _____

surgical removal of   means _____
the uterus   _____ ;

hysteropathy
his ter op´ ō thē   h _____
disease of the   means _____
uterus   _____ .

26.
Try it again using the word roots metr, metr/o. Build a term and then write its meaning:

-scope   -itis
-atrophy (wasting away, diminishing in size)

metroscope
mēt´ rō skōp   M _____
instrument for   means _____
examining the   _____ ;
uterus
metritis mē trī´ tis   m _____
inflammation of   means _____
uterine tissues   _____ ;
metratrophy
mē trat´ rō fē   m _____
uterine tissue   means _____
atrophy   _____ .

27.
Use the word roots metr/, metr/o with the following suffixes to make a new word that fits each of the definitions:

     -orrhagia means hemorrhage
     -orrhea means flow or discharge

metrorrhagia
mē trō rā´ jē ə
metrorrhea
mē trō rē´ ə

uterine hemorrhage _____ ;
discharge from the uterus (mucus or pus)

_____ .

28.
Here are two suffixes that can be confusing:

     -orrhexis means rupture (bursting open);
     -ocele means hernia or rupture.

The difference between them is the degree of severity of the outcome; the first has a high mortality.

hysterorrhexis
his´ ter ō rek´ sis

Build a term meaning ruptured uterus (ruptured during labor threatening the mother's life and perhaps the infant's):
hyster_____ .

hysterocele
his´ ter ō sēl

Build a term meaning uterine hernia (to be repaired by a surgeon):
hyster_____ .

29.
Endo/metr/ium refers to the inside lining of the uterus. Myo/metr/ium refers to the muscle layer of the uterus.

endo/myo/metr/itis
en dō mī ō mē
trī´ tis

Build a term meaning inflammation of the inside lining and muscle layers of the uterus:

_____ / _____ / _____ / _____ .
inside   muscle   uterus   inflammation

hyster, hyster/o metr, metr/o	**30.** Two word roots refer to the uterus. They are _____ and _____.
hyster/o metr/o	**31.** The term meaning the whole organ is _____. The term referring to the tissues of the organ is _____.
menstruation men strū ā′ shun	**32.** Now let's look at a uterine function. Menses, men/o means monthly flow of bloody fluid from the uterus. Menstruation is the function of discharging the menses. Men/o in any word should make you think of _____.
dis men ō rē′ a difficult or painful menstruation	**33.** Men/o/rrhea means free flow of menses, also known as menstruation. Dys/men/o/rrhea means _____.
me nor al′ jē a painful menstruation	**34.** Men/o/rrh/algia also means _____ _____.

men ō mē trō rā′
  jē ə
excessive bleeding
  (hemorrhage)
  from the uterus
  during
  menstruation
	35.
	Try this.
	Men/o/metr/o/rrhagia means _____
	_____
	_____.

menses men′ sēs	**36.** Menopause is a normal physiological condition of a mature woman. It's an event that ends a woman's menstrual life. This event marks the end of her childbearing period. It means the permanent cessation of _____.

children

37.
Menopause means the permanent cessation of the menses. It marks the end of a woman's capability for bearing _____.

cessation of
menses, or
menopause

38.
Climacteric is a transitional period of life sometimes called the change of life. It is a period between ages 45 and 60 when many changes take place in a woman's body. At the end of this transitional period, she no longer experiences menstruation and is no longer capable of bearing a child. The outcome of this transitional period is

_____.

climacteric
klī mak´ ter ik

39.
The critical period of life marking the beginning of the end of childbearing and ending with the onset of menopause is called the _____.

40.
During the female climacteric a key physical change takes place. The ovaries permanently and irreversibly atrophy. The production of estogen and progesterone declines, bringing an end of the reproductive period.

climacteric
complete cessation
of menses

This transitional period of life is called the _____. The outcome of this transition period is the menopause, which means

_____.

climacteric

41.
Men also experience a decline in sexual activity in their presenile years. This change of life period in a man is called the male _____.

climacteric

42.
Menopause ends the body's reproductive function. What word describes the transitional period of critical changes that ends in menopause?

_____.

43.
It's time to review the word combinations you've learned in this section. From the suggested answers, select a term to go with each definition. Write your selection in the space provided.

hysteropathy   mammography
mastodynia   gynecomastia
metrorrhagia   endometritis

woman's breast (in a male),

gynecomastia   _____.
hysteropathy   uterine disease, _____.
mastodynia   painful breast, _____.
                inflammation inside the uterus,
endometritis   _____.
                X ray examination of the breast,
mammography   _____.
                uterine hemorrhage,
metrorrhagia   _____.

44.
Here are a few more.

SUGGESTED ANSWERS:

hysterorrhexis   menorrhalgia
amenorrhea   climactric (female)
menopause   metratrophy

permanent cessation of menses,

menopause   _____.

                lack of menstruation (temporary),

amenorrhea   _____.

                rupture of uterus (during labor),

hysterorrhexis _____.

                change of life transition period,

climacteric   _____.
   (female)
menorrhalgia   painful menstruation,

                _____.

                wasting (diminishing in size) of the uterus,

metratrophy   _____.

Pregnancy and Childbirth

In this section you'll learn one term at a time. First you'll read a brief paragraph defining the new term. Then you'll answer questions and complete statements about it showing you understand what it means.

Read the following paragraph about conception. Then complete frames 45 to 47. Feel free to refer back to the paragraph as you work through the frames.

Conception means fertilization. It's an event marked by penetration of the ovum (female egg cell) by a spermatozoon (male germ cell). Conception results in a fertilized ovum. Only a fertilized ovum develops into a human being.

fertilization or
conception

45.
Penetration of the female egg cell by the male germ cell is known as _____.

ovum

spermatozoon

46.
Another term for female egg cell is
_____.
A term meaning male germ cell is
_____.

conception

fertilized

47.
Union of an ovum and a spermatozoon is called
_____.
A child will develop from an ovum only if the ovum is _____.

Gestation is the period from conception to childbirth during which an ovum passes through several stages of development on the way to becoming a newborn infant. Gestation lasts approximately 9 months, or 280 days from the last menstrual period.

48.
Gestation is another word for

pregnancy
gestation
jes tā´ shun

_____.

Pregnancy is another word for

_____.

49.
Gestation is the process of developing an ovum

9

280

into a child. It takes approximately _____ months, or _____ days.

50.
An ovum develops into a child during a period

gestation
pregnancy

from conception to birth. This process is called _____ or _____.

51.
During pregnancy an ovum passes through a couple of developmental stages or phases. Taken together, these phases make up the nine-month

gestation

period called _____.

The earliest gestational phase begins with a fertilized female egg cell. In just two weeks, the ovum divides into two cells, and each cell continues halving until it has become a complex mass of cells. This mass of cells is now called an embryo. It's a living organism ready to continue its development in the next phase.

52.
The indispensable event that initiates pregnancy is

conception   _____.

53.
ovum
ō´ vum   After conception, the earliest phase of development
two   begins with a fertilized _____ and
lasts _____ weeks.

54.
The first two weeks of gestation produces a
embryo   complex living organism called a/an
em´ brē ō
_____.

An embryo begins the second stage of gestation,
which lasts six weeks. In the third week, the
embryo begins to acquire structure (head, arms,
legs, and a tail), and over the next few weeks it
begins forming principal internal organs and body
systems. By the end of the eighth week of gestation
the embryo looks somewhat like a human and is
called a fetus.

55.
The second stage of gestation begins with a two-
week-old ovum, which is now called an
embryo   _____.

56.
An embryo begins its development in the
third   _____ week of gestation and
eighth   continues through the _____
week of a new pregnancy.

57.
During this second gestational phase the embryo
begins forming arms and legs and principal
organs   internal _____.

58.

By the beginning of the ninth week, the embryo is beginning to resemble a

human being

fetus

fē´ tus

_____ and is called a

_____.

A fetus begins the last phase of gestation. A fetus is a live offspring while it is in the mother (in utero). It develops into a viable child during the remainder of the gestational period. The fetal stage lasts from the beginning of the third month of gestation to childbirth.

59.

In the last gestational phase, the fetus in utero

viable child

at three months

   pregnant

seven months

childbirth

develops into a _____.

When does this phase begin? _____

_____.

How long does it last? _____.

What is the terminating event?

_____.

60.

Here's a quick review.

• Penetration of an ovum by a spermatozoon is

conception

called _____.

• A nine-month period during which a fertilized ovum becomes a child is called

gestation

_____.

• In the first two weeks of pregnancy an ovum becomes a complex organism called an

embryo

_____.

• From the third week to the beginning of the ninth week of pregnancy an embryo develops rudimentary appendages and internal

organs

_____.

• After only two months´ gestation, the embryo

a human being

fetus

begins to resemble _____ and is

called a _____ .

human being or

   child

childbirth

• A fetus developing in utero for the next seven months becomes a _____.

• Gestation ends with _____.

Here are a few medical terms referring to some structures and conditions relating to pregnancy. Amnion, amni/o, amniot/o refer to a thin transparent sac containing the fetus and the fluid surrounding the fetus. This sac grows rapidly as the fetus inside develops. The amniotic fluid protects the fetus from injury and helps maintain an even temperature.

61.
amniotic fluid
am nē ot´ ik flū´ id

Within the amniotic sac the fetus is protected from injury and changes in temperature by the *liquor amnii*, or in other words, _____

_____ .

62.
amniotic

Amniot/itis means inflammation of the amnion. Build a word meaning pertaining to the sac that envelops the fetus : _____ .

63.
am´ nē ō sen tē´ sis
puncturing the
  amniotic sac and
  withdrawing
  some fluid

Centesis is the suffix meaning to puncture a cavity and remove fluid. Explain the meaning of amni/o/centesis: _____

_____ .

64.
am´ nē ō tōm
X ray study of the
  amnion (and its
  contents)

Amni/o/tome is an instrument for cutting (puncturing) the amnion. What does amni/ography mean? _____

_____ .

65.
ol´ i gō hī dram´ nē
  os
scanty amount of
  amniotic fluid in
  the sac

Olig-, oligo- is a prefix meaning little, small, scanty. Olig/uria means scanty urination. What does oligo/hydr/amnios mean? _____

_____ .

66.
excessive amount
  of amniotic fluid
  in the sac

What do you think polyhydramnios means?

_____

_____ .

amniotic sac or
amnion

67.
What structure envelops the fetus and contains the fluid protecting the fetus? _____
_____.

Placenta is the vascular structure through which a fetus absorbs oxygen, nutrients, and other substances from its mother and excretes carbon dioxide and other wastes. It begins forming about the eighth day of gestation, and at the end of pregnancy weighs about one-sixth of the weight of the infant. The placenta makes an intimate connection with the inside lining of the uterus and is attached to the fetus by the umbilical cord. The placenta is expelled after the child is born and therefore is called the afterbirth.

placenta

68.
The fetus in utero absorbs oxygen and nutrients and excretes carbon dioxide and wastes through a vascular structure called the _____.

1 pound
1 ounce

69.
If the baby's birth weight is 6 pounds, 6 ounces, what would you expect the placenta to weigh at the end of pregnancy? _____ pound _____ ounce.

en dō mē´ trē um
the inside lining of
the uterus

70.
The placenta forms and grows on the endometrium and makes an intimate bond with it. What is the endometrium? _____
_____.

placenta

umbilical cord

71.
While in utero the fetus grows by getting its nourishment through the _____.
The fetus is attached to the placenta by the
_____.

72.

afterbirth

The placenta is expelled after the baby is born. The placenta is also called _____.

73.

pregnant

Gravida, gravid refers to a pregnant woman; being heavy with child. Gravidism is the condition of being _____.

prī´ ma grav´ i da
a woman who is
   pregnant with
   her first child
a woman in her
   second
   pregnancy
secundigravida
sē kun´ da grav´ i
   da

74.

Primi- means first; secundi- means second. Primigravida means _____
_____.

What do you think gravida II means?

_____
_____.

Build a term meaning a woman in her second pregnancy: _____.

75.

Here's a quick review. From the suggested answers, select a term to go with each definition. Write your selection in the space provided.

SUGGESTED ANSWERS:

oligohydramnios	primigravida
amniocentesis	secundigravida
amniotic fluid	placenta

secundigravida

a woman's second pregnancy,
_____.

primigravida

a pregnant woman, first time,
_____.

oligohydramnios

scanty fluid in the amnion,
_____.

placenta
amniotic fluid

fetus in utero absorbs nutrients and excretes waste through it, _____.
liquor amnii, _____.

amniocentesis

puncture of the amnion and removal of fluid,
_____.

Labor is the process by which a baby is born and the placenta expelled from the uterus. Labor has three stages. The first stage is the stage of dilation. It is characterized by contractions of the uterine muscle and dilation of the opening of the cervix—wide enough to let the baby out. The second stage is expulsion. The baby is born! The third is the afterbirth stage. The placenta is expelled. The average duration of labor is about 13 hours in first pregnancies (12 hours in the first stage, 1 hour in the second, few minutes in the third) and about 8 hours in subsequent pregnancies.

76.
At term, when gestation is completed, a three-stage physiological process begins. It is called

labor   _____.

77.
In the first stage of labor, the uterus contracts rhythmically for 8 to 12 hours. The cervix stretches and opens until it is fully dilated so the baby may
dilation   pass through the birth canal. This first stage is
dī lā´ shun   called the _____ stage.

78.
The second stage of labor involves expulsion. The infant passes through the birth canal and is

born   _____.

79.
Expulsion of the placenta follows the birth of the child. The expelled placenta is more commonly
afterbirth   known as the _____.

80.
What happens during the expulsion stage, or the second stage of labor? _____.

a child is born
   (expelled)

81.
How long is the third stage of labor?
_____.
What happens in the afterbirth stage of labor?
_____.

a few minutes
the placenta is
   expelled

82.
After 8 to 12 hours of uterine contractions during the first stage of labor, what has happened?
_____
_____.

the (neck of the)
   uterus
   completely
   dilates (opens)

83.
Parturition is another word for childbirth. What other term you just learned also means the act of being born? _____.

par tyer ish´ un

labor

84.
Antepartum means the period of time before labor begins.

What does postpartum mean? _____
_____.

pertaining to after
   labor

85.
Neo means new or recent. *Natus* is a Latin term for birth. What does neonatal mean?
_____
_____.

pertaining to the
   recent period
   around
   childbirth

pertaining to medical care and supervision of a pregnant woman before childbirth	**86.** What do you think prenatal care means? _____ _____.

87.
Review the terms you just learned before moving on. Select the term that best fits each brief definition. Use the suggestions if you need help.

labor   parturition
prenatal care   afterbirth
dilation   expulsion

prenatal care
prē nā´ tal kair

labor

parturition

dilation

expulsion

afterbirth

medical supervision of a pregnant woman,
_____.

the process of giving birth,
_____.

the act of childbirth,
_____.

first stage of labor,
_____.

second stage of labor,
_____.

third stage of labor,
_____.

88.
Pudendum, pudenda (plural) means the external genitals (sex organs) of a female. (These parts are easily observed without manual examination. They include the clitoris, vulva, and entrance of the vagina.) Refer to the illustrations in frame 19.

pudenda
pyōō den´ də

Build a term meaning pertaining to the female's external genitals: _____.

89.

Perineum refers to the structures that make up the pelvic outlet and comprise the pelvic floor. It is the region between the vulva and anus in a female or between the scrotum and _____ in a male.

anus
ā´ nus

90.

A baby coming through the birth canal during parturition can overstretch the vagina and the pelvic outlet. A tear (laceration) may occur in the tissues around the pelvic outlet. This pelvic floor structure is called the _____.

perineum
per i nē´ um

Episiotomy is an incision of the perineum. In the second stage of labor, just before the baby is born, the obstetrician may incise the perineum to avoid a more damaging laceration of the surrounding tissues.

91.

An incision into the perineum is called

_____.

episiotomy
e pēz ē ot´ ō mē

92.

Episiotomy controls damage to the tissues of the vagina and _____.

perineum

repair, recon-
    struction of the
    tissues after an
    episiotomy

93.

What does episiorrhaphy mean?

_____

_____.

Here's a term often confused with perineum. Peritoneum is a tough membrane covering the viscera (organs in the belly) and lining the abdominal cavity. It clings to the viscera as plastic wrap clings to whatever it covers.

peritoneum
per i tō nē´ um

per i tō nī´ tis
inflammation of
   the peritoneum

94.
The membrane coating the viscera and lining the abdominal cavity is the _____.

What is peritonitis? _____
_____.

95.
Select one of the terms that best fits the brief definition. Write it in the space provided.

peritoneum   episiotomy
pudenda   perineum

perineum

pudenda

peritoneum

episiotomy

area between the vulva and anus,
_____.
external female genitals, _____.
membrane coating viscera and lining abdominal wall, _____.
incision of the perineum limiting injury of the pelvic outlet during childbirth,
_____.

Involution is the process that reduces the uterus to its normal nonpregnant size and condition following childbirth.

involution
in vō lū´ shun

96.
The process that returns an enlarged uterus to its normal size is called _____.

Puerperium is the period following the third stage of labor, when involution takes place. Involution lasts approximately six weeks.

poo er pĕr´ ē um
expelled

97.
Puerperium begins after the fetus and the placenta have been _____.

six

98.
Puerperium lasts until the uterus returns to its size and condition before pregnancy began. This period is approximately _____ weeks.

involution

99.
After fulfilling its function, the uterus goes through a process of returning to its earlier nonpregnant condition. This process is called

_____.

puerperium
poo er pĕr´ ē um

100.
Involution takes place during a six-week period after childbirth. This period is called

_____.

puerper/al
poo er´ per al

101.
Build a term meaning pertaining to the period after childbirth when involution takes place:
_____/_____.

puerperal

102.
Prior to effective antibiotic therapy the greatest single cause of death following childbirth was childbed fever. It is an infection of the genital tract occurring during the puerperium called
_____ sepsis.

inflammation of
  the peritoneum
  during
  puerperium

103.
What is puerperal peritonitis?
_____
_____.

the uterus returns
   to its earlier
   nonpregnant
   state after
   childbirth

104.
Involution takes place during puerperium. What
does involution mean? _____
_____
_____.

nulli/para
nullipara
nu lip′ ə ra

105.
Nulli- is a prefix meaning none. Para means to bear
a child. Build a term that refers to a woman who
has never born a child: _____/_____.

prīm ip′ ə ra
a woman who has
   given birth to
   one viable child

106.
A woman who has delivered more than one living
child is described as multipara. What does
primipara mean? _____
_____.

she has given birth
   to two viable
   children

107.
What does an obstetrician mean when he writes in
the patient's chart that she is para-2? _____
_____.

primipara
nullipara
multipara
mul tip′ ə ra

108.
Using the word root para and nulli-, multi-, or
primi-, build a word for each of the following
abbreviations.
para-1, _____.
para-0, _____.
para-4, _____.

109.

It's a good time to review what you just covered. Select a term from the suggestions and complete each brief definition.

nullipara   parturition
primigravida   antepartum
involution   puerperium

process that reduces the uterus to normal size and condition after childbirth,

involution

_____.

six-week period after childbirth when involution

puerperium   takes place, _____.

period in pregnancy before labor,

antepartum

_____.

woman who has never given birth to a viable child,

nullipara

_____.

a woman who is pregnant for the first time ever,

primigravida

_____.

another term for labor,

parturition

_____.

110.

Here are some terms you may find very interesting. Look them up in your medical dictionary. You'll be surprised at how much you have learned.

acquired   congenital
anomaly   eclampsia
placenta abruptio   placenta previa

111.

Here are 48 new words you worked with in this unit. When you pronounce each term be sure to think about what it means. Then take the Unit 8 Self-Test.

amenorrhea (ä men ō rē′ a)

amniocentesis (am′ nē ō sen tē′ sis)

amnion (am′ nē on)

amniotic fluid (am nē ôt ik flōō′ id)

climacteric (klī mak′ ter ik)

conception (kon sep′ shun)

dysmenorrhea (dis men ōr ē′ ə)

embryo

endometrium (en′ dō mē′ trē um)

episiotomy (e pēz ē ot′ ō mē)

fetus

gestation (jes tā′ shun)

gynecomastia (gī′ ne kō mas′ tē ə)

gynoplasty (jin′ ō plas tē)

hysterocele (his′ ter ō sēl)

hysteromyoma (his′ ter ō mī ō′ mä)

hysterorrhexis (his′ ter ō rek′ sis)

involution (in vō lōō′ shun)

labor

mammalgia (ma mal′ jē ə)

mammary (mam′ ə rē)

mammopexy (mam′ ō pek sē)

mastodynia (mas tō din′ ē ə)

mastoncus (mas tong′ kus)

mastopathy (mas top′ ə thē)

mastoptosis (mas top tō′ sis)

menometrorrhagia (men′ ō mētrō rā′ jē ə)

menopause (men′ ō pawz)

menorrhalgia (men ō ral′ jē ə)

menses (men′ sēz)

menstruation (men strū ā′ shun)

metratrophy (mē trat′ rō fē)

multipara (mul tip′ ə ra)

myometritis (mī′ ō mē trī′ tis)

neonatal (nē ō nā′ tal)

nullipara (nu lip′ ə ra)

oligohydramnios (ol′ ē gō hī dram′ nē ōs)

ovum (ō′ vum)

parturition (pär tyōōr ish′ un)

perineum (per i nē′ um)

peritoneum (per i tō nē′ um)

placenta

postpartum

primigravida (prī′ ma grav′ i da)

pudenda (pyōō den′ də)

puerperal sepsis (pōō er′ per al sep sis)

puerperium (pōō er pēr′ ē um)

spermatozoon (sper′ ma tō zō′ on)

Unit 8 Self-Test

PART 1

From the right, select the correct meaning for each of the following medical terms.

_____ 1. Primigravida
_____ 2. Pudenda
_____ 3. Hysteropathy
_____ 4. Mammary
_____ 5. Mastrodynia
_____ 6. Amniotic
_____ 7. Episiotomy
_____ 8. Endometritis
_____ 9. Involution
_____ 10. Metratrophy
_____ 11. Perineum
_____ 12. Amenorrhea
_____ 13. Puerperium
_____ 14. Hysterorrhexis
_____ 15. Mammography

a. X ray study of the breast
b. Temporary lack of menstruation
c. Pelvic floor, region from vulva to anus
d. Process returning uterus to nonpregnant state
e. Incision of vagina and pelvic outlet
f. Female external genitals
g. Pregnant woman, first time
h. Period after childbirth, when involution takes place
i. Pertaining to sac holding the fetus and fluid
j. Rupture of uterus (during labor)
k. Pertaining to the breast
l. Uterine atrophy (wasting)
m. Inflammation of uterine inside lining
n. Painful breasts
o. Uterine disease

PART 2

Write the medical term for each of the following brief definitions.

1. Surgical fixation of pendulus breasts   Mammo _____
2. Membrane covering abdominal viscera   Peri _____
3. Painful breasts   _____ dynia

4. Change of life period   Female _____

5. Organism in utero resembling
   a human   _____

6. Organ that nourishes fetus
   in utero   Pl_____

7. Surgical removal of the breast   _____

8. Another term for pregnancy   G_____

9. Pertaining to a recently born
   child   _____

10. Woman pregnant with her first
    child   _____

11. Pendulous breast   _____

12. Fertilization of an ovum   C_____

13. Labor and delivery of term
    pregnancy   Part_____

14. Before the onset of labor   Ante_____

15. After childbirth when
    involution takes place   Puer_____

ANSWERS

Part 1

1. g	9. d
2. f	10. l
3. o	11. c
4. k	12. b
5. n	13. h
6. i	14. j
7. e	15. a
8. m	

Part 2

1. Mammopexy	9. Neonatal
2. Peritoneum	10. Primipara
3. Mastodynia	11. Mastoptosis
4. Female climacteric	12. Conception
5. Fetus	13. Parturition
6. Placenta	14. Antepartum
7. Mastectomy	15. Puerperium
8. Gestation	

Unit 9

In this final unit you will form medical terms relating to the eye and the respiratory system. Some of the new word roots and prefixes you will use are as follows:

blephar/o (*eyelid*)
core, core/o (*pupil*)
corne/o, kerat/o (*cornea*)
cycl/o (*ciliary body*)
dipl/o (*paired, double*)
ir, irid/o (*iris*)
lacrim/o (*tear*)
ophthalm/o (*eye*)
retin/o (*retina*)
scler/o (*sclera*)

bronch/i (*bronch/o, bronchus*)
laryng/o (*voice box*)
ment/o (*chin*)
nas/o (*nose*)
pharyng/o (*throat*)
pleur/o (*covering of the lung*)
pneum/o (*air, breathe*)
pneumon/o (*lung*)
thorac/o (*thorax*)
trache/o (*windpipe*)

The Eye

1.
Ophthalmology is the medical specialty concerned with the eye, its diseases, and refractive errors. Ophthalm/o/malacia means an abnormal softening of the eyeball. Ophthalm/ic means

relating to the eye   _____.

2.
Ophthalm, ophthalm/o are word roots that are difficult to spell and pronounce. But if you pronounce the words correctly, the spelling will be easier. For example, oph thal mo is pronounced

of   of thal´ mō. The oph is pronounced as _____.
In the word root ophthalm-, ph comes before th.

of thal´ mō   Oph thal mō is pronounced _____.

                        Pronounce it.

3.
Here's a chance to practice your spelling and pronunciation. Use the word root ophthalm/o and add each of these suffixes to build new words.
    -cele (hernia, herniation)
    -meter (instrument for measuring)
    -plegia (paralysis)
Build a term and then pronounce it carefully:

ophthalmocele   herniation of the eye (abnormal protrusion),
of thal´ mō sēl   _____;

ophthalmometer   instrument for measuring the eye,
of´ thal mō´ meter   _____;

ophthalmoplegia   paralysis of the eye,
of thal´ mo plē´ gē a   _____.

4.
The physician who practices the medical specialty concerned with diseases of the eye is an

ophthalmologist
of thal mol´ ō jist   _____.

5.
The instrument used for studying the interior of the eyeball through the pupil is an

ophthalmoscope
of thal´ mō skōp

_____.

6.
Dipl/o means double or paired. Opia is a word root meaning vision. What does dipl/opia mean?

double vision

_____.

7.
Whenever a pair of eyes fail to record the same image on the brain, a double image occurs. The medical term for double vision is

diplopia
di plō´ pē a

_____.

8.
Write a brief meaning for each of the following.

double (or paired)
    bacteria
bluish vision

dipl/o/bacteria, _____
_____;
cyan/opia; _____.

9.
Blephar/optosis means prolapse (drooping) of an eyelid. The word root for eyelid is

blef a rop´ tō sis
blephar- blephar/o

_____.

10.
Blephar/edema means fluid in the tissues of the eyelid. Underline the part of the term meaning swelling due to fluid in the tissues: blepharedema.

blef ar e dē´ ma
blephar<u>edema</u>

11.
The condition of swollen eyelids due to edema is

blepharedema

_____.

12.

blef´ ar ō spazm
twitching of the
   eyelid
blef ar ōr´ a fē
suturing of the
   eyelid

Define each of the following terms:

blepharospasm means _____
_____.

blepharorrhaphy means _____
_____.

13.

blef ar ī´ tis
blepharitis

Build a word that means inflammation of the
eyelid, _____.

The Eye

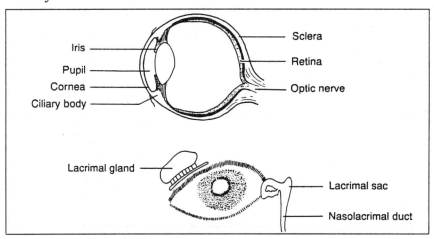

Iris
Pupil
Cornea
Ciliary body

Sclera
Retina
Optic nerve

Lacrimal gland

Lacrimal sac
Nasolacrimal duct

14.
Use the illustration to help you work through
frames 15 to 38.

15.

kor nē al
pertaining to the
   cornea
ker a top´ a thē
disease of the
   cornea

The cornea is the transparent tissue covering the
anterior sixth of the eye. Kerat, kerat/o form words
referring to the cornea. Write the meaning of each
of the following:
corneal _____;
kerat/o/pathy _____.

16.
Using the word root kerat/o, build a term meaning plastic repair of the cornea:

keratoplasty
ker´ a tō plas tē
_____.

17.
The cornea is one-sixth of the outer coat of the eyeball. It is the transparent tissue covering the front of the eyeball. The word root meaning cornea

kerat, kerat/o
is _____.

18.
Scler/o refers to the white of the eye. The sclera is the hard fibrous coat forming the outer envelope of the eye. It covers five-sixths of the eyeball. The other anterior sixth is occupied by the

cornea
_____.

19.
Corneoscleral means pertaining to an area where the cornea meets the sclera. Write the meaning for each of the following:

skler´ al
pertaining to the
    sclera
scleral _____

skler´ ō tōm
_____;

instrument for
    cutting the sclera
sclerotome _____
_____.

20.
Sclerectasia means bulging (stretching) of the white of the eye. Build a term meaning excision of a portion of the sclera:

sclerectomy
skle rek´ tō mē
_____.

ī´ ris
ir´ i dō kor´ nē al
pertaining to the
   area where the
   iris and cornea
   meet
ir´ id ō sēl
hernia of the iris

21.
Iris means rainbow. The iris is a diaphragm
perforated in the center (the pupil). The word roots
referring to the donut-shaped color in the eye are ir,
irid, and irid/o. What do you think iridocorneal
means? _____

_____

Iridocele means _____

_____

ir/itus
iritis
ī rī´ tis

22.
One of the word roots for the iris is ir. It has very
limited use, but it's always used to express
inflammation.
Using the word root ir build a word meaning
inflammation of the iris: _____/_____.

i ri dal´ jē ə
pain in the iris

23.
Irid/o is the word root used to refer to the iris in
almost all other words. Iridalgia means

_____.

iridectomy
i ri dek´ tō mē

24.
Build a term meaning excision of part of the iris:

_____.

cornea
iris
iris
scelera
eye
eyelid

25.
Write what each of the following word roots
means.
kerat/o, _____.
ir, _____.
irid/o, _____.
scler/o, _____.
ophthalm/o, _____.
blephar/o, _____.

26.
Retin/o refers to the complex membrane lining the inside back surface of the eye. It receives the visual light rays which the brain interprets and gives meaning. Build a word meaning

retinal
ret´ i n'l
retinitis
ret i nī´ tis
retinoid
ret´ i noyd

pertaining to the retina, _____;
inflammation of the retina, _____;
resembling the retina, _____.

27.
Retinopexy means affixing (or adhering) the retina to the wall of the eyeball for correcting retinal detachment. What would you call an instrument for examining the retina to look for retinopathy?

retinoscope or
    ophthalmoscope
ret´ i nō skōp

_____.

ret i nop´ a thē
disease of the
    retina

28.
What does retinopathy mean? _____
_____.

29.
The pupil is the circular opening in the center of the iris through which the light rays enter the eye. It is the core or center of the eye. Cor, core/o refer to the pupil in the center of the

eye

30.
Cor/ectasia means dilation (stretching) of the pupil. What does cor/ectopia mean? _____

kōr ek tō´ pē a
a misplaced pupil

_____.

31.
Coreoplasty is a surgical procedure for correcting a deformed pupil. Write a meaning for coreometry:

kōr ē om´ e trē
measuring the size
    of a pupil

_____.

32.
Take another look at the illustration of the eye. The ciliary body controls a circular muscle that adjusts the shape of the lens. The word root for ciliary body is cycl/o. It means circle or surrounding. What does cyclo/paralysis mean? _____

_____

sī klō pa ral´ i sis
paralysis of the
    ciliary body

33.
Cyclocryotherapy means freezing of the ciliary body in the treatment of glaucoma. Underline the part of the term referring to freezing: cyclocryotherapy.

sī klō krī´ ō ther´
    a pē
cyclo<u>cryo</u>therapy

34.
Cyclitis means inflammation of the ciliary body. What is the meaning of cyclokeratitis?

_____

_____.

sī klō ker a tī´ tis
inflammation of
    the cornea and
    the ciliary body

35.
Look again at the illustration. The lacrimal apparatus consists of the gland, the sac, and the duct. The purpose of the lacrimal apparatus is to keep the surface of the eye moist. What do you think lacrimal means?

_____.

lak´ ri mal
relating to tears

36.
The gland that secretes tears is the
_____ gland.
The sac that collects the tears is the
_____ sac.

lacrimal

lacrimal

37.
What is the structure that empties the tears into the nasal cavity? _____ _____.

nasolacrimal duct

38.

Tears keep the surface of the eye moistened. Tears are continually being formed and removed. When tears form more quickly than they can be removed by the lacrimal apparatus, we say the person is

crying _____.

39.

How about a review. Complete each of the following brief definitions. Use the suggested answers to help you.

SUGGESTED ANSWERS:

iritis	cycloplegia
lacrimal	sclerotome
retinoscopy	ophthalmic
coreometry	keratitis
iridocele	keratoplasty

measurement of pupil size,

coreometry _____.

herniation of the iris,

iridocele _____.

pertaining to the eye,

ophthalmic _____.

examination of the retina,

retinoscopy _____.

inflammation of the iris,

iritis _____.

instrument for cutting the sclera,

sclerotome _____.

relating to tears,

lacrimal _____.

surgical reconstruction of the cornea,

keratoplasty _____.

paralytic ciliary body,

cycloplegia _____.

inflammation of the cornea,

keratitis _____.

40.

Try these now. Write the meaning of each of the following word roots:

retina

pupil

ciliary body

eyelid

cornea

eye

retin/o, _____.

cor/o, core/o, _____.

cycl/o, _____.

blephar/o, _____.

kerat/o (corne/o), _____.

ophthalm/o, _____.

The Respiratory System

41.

Use the illustration and table to work frames 42 to 85. If you have forgotten a word root, remember you may look back. If you don't know the anatomy of the respiratory system, look at the diagram provided for you. Seeing the parts as you work will make your learning more interesting.

The Respiratory System

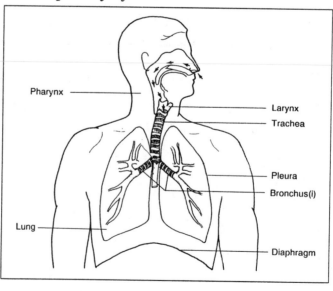

Word Roots for Anatomical Terms

nas/o	(*nose*)
pharynx	(*throat*)
larynx	(*voice box*)
trachea	(*windpipe*)
bronchus	(*one of two main branches of the windpipe*)
pleura	(*a tough, wet, and slippery thin film covering the lungs*)
diaphragm	(*a musculomembranous wall separating the abdomen from the thoracic cavity*)

42.

Ment, ment/o means chin. Nas/o/ment/al means

nose

nasal

nā z'l

pertaining to the chin and _____

Build a term meaning pertaining to the nose:

_____ .

43.

Analyze the term nasomental.

nas/o

ment/o

al

The word root for nose is _____ .

The word root for chin is _____ .

The ending meaning pertaining to is _____ .

44.

Refer to the table in frame 41 to help you identify the word root for each anatomical part:

la rin jī´ tis

inflammation of
   the voice box

plōōr ī´ tis

inflammation of
   the pleura

fair ing´ gō plas tē

plastic surgery of
   the throat

laryng/itis means _____

_____

pleuritis means _____

_____ ;

pharyng/o/plasty means _____

_____ .

45.

Look again at the table. Cele means herniation of.

la ring´ gō sēl

herniation of the
   voice box

What does laryng /o/cele mean?

_____

_____ .

laryngectomy
la rin jek´ tō mē

46.
Build a term meaning surgical removal of the voice box: _____.

la ring´ gō skōp
instrument for
   examining the
   voice box
la ring´ gō spazm
spasm of the voice
  box

47.
Write a meaning for each of the following:

laryngoscope means _____
_____.

laryngospasm means _____
_____.

trā kē ō rā´ jē ə
hemorrhage from
   the windpipe
trā kē al´ jē ə
pain in the
   windpipe
trā kē os´ tō mē
a permanent
   opening into the
   windpipe

48.
Trachea means windpipe. Write a brief definition for each of the following new terms:

tracheorrhagia _____
_____.

trachealgia _____
_____.

trachesostomy _____
_____.

trach or trache/o

49.
Write the word root for windpipe:
_____.

brong kos´ kō pē
looking into the
   bronchus
bron´ kō spazm
spasm of the
   bronchus
brong kī´ tis
inflammation of
   the bronchus or
   bronchi

50.
A bronchus is one of the major divisions of the windpipe. The bronchi (plural) direct the air into the lungs. Write a meaning for each of the following:

bronchoscopy _____
_____.

bronchospasm _____
_____.

bronchitis _____
_____.

51.
The word root meaning major branches of the windpipe that open into the lungs is

bronch, or
bronch/o

_____.

52.
Pleural means pertaining to the covering on the lungs. The pleural membrane completely covers the lungs and clings to it like plastic wrap. Only a few drops of thick fluid keep the lung and the pleura apart.

plōō rī´ tis
inflammation of
the pleura

Pleuritis means _____

_____.

pleuralgia or
pleurdynia
plōō ral´ jē ə
plōō rō din´ ē ə

53.
Pleurisy is another word for inflammation of the covering of the lungs. Build a term that means pain in the pleura: _____.

plōō rō sen tē´ sis
puncture of the
pleural space
and removing
the fluid

54.
Pleurisy may cause excessive fluid to collect within the space between the lung and the pleura. What do you think pleurocentesis means?

_____

_____.

diaphragm
dī´ a fram

55.
Refer to the illustration in frame 41 again. The musculomembranous wall separating the abdomen from the chest cavity is the _____.

in

56.
During inspiration the diaphragm contracts; it flattens out downward, permitting the lungs to move downward and fill with air. Inspiration is breathing _____.
(in / out)

57.
During expiration the diaphragm relaxes. It resumes its inverted basin shape, squeezing the lungs and expelling the air out of the lungs. Expiration is breathing _____.
                                        (in / out)

out

58.
The organ responsible for inspiration and expiration is the _____.

diaphragm

59.
A sudden spasm of the diaphragm usually produces a giggle all around. It is called singultus . Can you guess what it means?
_____.

hiccough, or
  hiccup
hik´ kof

60.
Another term for hiccup is
_____.

singultus
sin gul´ tus

61.
Ptysis means spitting. What does hem/o/ptysis mean? _____.

hē mop´ ti sis
spitting blood

62.
Hemoptysis means spitting blood arising from hemorrhage of larynx, trachea, bronchi, or lungs. What does hemat/emesis mean? _____
_____.

hē ma tem´ a sis
expelling blood
  from the
  stomach

63.
Write two combining forms for blood:
_____ and _____.

hem/o, hemat/o

64.
Spitting blood from hemorrhage of the lungs is
_____. Expelling blood
from the stomach is _____.

hemoptysis
hematemesis

65.
Epistaxis means hemorrhage from the nose. What
does rhinorrhagia mean? _____
_____.

rīn or ra´ jē a
hemorrhage from
    the nose

66.
Two terms mean severe bleeding from the nose.
They are _____ and
_____.

epistaxis
ep i stak´ sis
rhinorrhagia

67.
What does hemoptysis mean?
_____
_____.

spitting blood
    (arising from the
    larynx, trachea,
    bronchi, or
    lungs)

68.
What does hematemesis mean?
_____
_____.

expelling blood
    from the
    stomach

69.
Nasal hemorrhage is _____ or
_____.

epistaxis
rhinorrhagia

70.
Pneum/o, pneumat/o mean air, gases, or exchange
of gases. What does pneumatic mean?
_____
_____.

nyo͞o mat´ ik
pertaining to air or
    gases (or ex-
    change of gases)

71.

brad ip nē´ a
breathing very
  slowly

Pne/o relates to breathing. Do you remember what
bradypnea means? _____
_____.

72.

pne/o (nē ō)
pneum/o or
  pneumat/o

The word root referring to inhale and exhale, or in
other words to breathe, is _____.
Write the word root referring to air or gases:
_____.

73.

nyōo mol´ ō jē
air or gases
not breathing
  (breathless)

Pneum/ology refers to the science of how the lungs
exchange _____ or _____.
Apnea means _____.

74.

pneumotherapy
nyōo mō ther´ ə pē

Hydrotherapy means treatment with water. Build a
term meaning treatment with (compressed) air:
_____.

75.

pneum/o
pneumat/o

pneumon/o

Pneumon, pneumon/o means lung. At a quick
glance you may confuse it with the root for air or
gases. Write them both: _____;
air or gases

_____.
lung

76.

pneumonitis
nyōo mō nī´ tis
pneumonectomy
nyōo mōn ek´ tō mē

Pneumonia is a serious disease of the lung. Build a
term for each of the following:
inflammation of the lung
_____.

surgical removal of a lung
_____.

77.
Drawing air into the lungs and pushing air out of the lungs is called breathing. The word root referring to breathing is _____.

pne/o (nē ō)

78.
Pneum/o/encephal/o/graphy means X ray examination of spaces within the brain. These X rays are taken following withdrawal of cerebrospinal fluid (via lumbar puncture) and replacement of it with injected air or gas. What is a pneumon/o/graph? _____
_____.

nyōō mon´ ō graf
radiographic
   picture of the
   lungs (chest
   X ray)

79.
Write a brief meaning for each of the following:
Pne/o _____.
Pneum/o or pneumat/o _____.
Pneumon/o _____.

breathing
air or gas
lung

80.
Thorax is the chest. It refers to the upper part of the trunk between the neck and the abdomen. The diaphragm separates the abdomen from the
_____.

thorax
thor´ aks

81.
The organs of the digestive apparatus are enclosed in the abdomen. The chief organs of the circulatory and respiratory systems are located in the
_____.

thorax

82.
Thorac and thorac/o are the word roots referring to the chest.
Thoracotomy means _____
_____.
Explain thoracocentesis: _____
_____.

thor a cot´ ə mē
incision into the
   chest
thor a cō sen tē´ sis
puncture of the
   chest to draw off
   fluid

83.
Pneumothorax means air in the chest. What does hemothorax mean? _____
_____.

hē mō thor´ aks
blood in the chest

84.
Let's conclude this unit with a review. Using the suggested answers, complete each of the following brief definitions. Write your answer in the space provided.

SUGGESTED ANSWERS:

bronchus(i)	pleura
diaphragm	trachea
larynx	singultus
pharynx	epistaxis

larynx   voice box, _____.
                  main branches of the windpipe,

bronchi   _____.

epistaxis   severe nosebleed _____.

trachea   windpipe, _____.

singultus   hiccup, _____.

pharynx   throat, _____.
                  tough film enveloping the lungs,

pleura   _____.
                  muscle controlling breathing,

diaphragm   _____.

85.
Try that again.

SUGGESTED ANSWERS:

apneic	hemoptysis
pneumothorax	rhinoplasty
pneumonogram	pneumonia
nasal	pleurodynia

                  serious lung condition,

pneumonia   _____.
                  spitting blood (arising from trachea),

hemoptysis   _____.

pneumonogram   X ray of the lung(s), _____.
                  collection of air in the chest,

pneumothorax   _____.

nasal   pertaining to the nose, _____.

rhinoplasty   a "nose job," _____.

pleurodynia   pain in the pleura, _____.
                  pertaining to breathlessness,

apneic   _____.

86.

Here's one last exercise to show how far you have come! For each area of medical concern, write the term describing a practicing specialist

	Area of Medical Concern	Specialist
	Nature, structure, and causes of disease	_____
Pathologist		
Psychiatrist	Mental illness	_____
Dermatologist	Skin and its diseases	_____
Gynecologist	Diseases of women	_____
Cardiologist	Diseases of the heart	_____
Neurologist	Nervous system diseases	_____
Pediatrician	Childhood illnesses	_____
Obstetrician	Pregnancy and childbirth	_____
Ophthalmologist	Diseases of the eye	_____
Urologist	Conditions of urogenitals	_____

87.

Try it again. Describe the area of medical concern for these specialists.

	Specialist	Area of Medical Concern
Bones and muscles	Orthopedist	_____
Pregnancy and childbirth	Obstetrician	_____
Old age, aging	Geriatrician	_____
Causes of epidemics	Epidemiologist	_____
Skilled diagnosing	Diagnostician	_____
Anesthesia and pain	Anesthesiologist	_____
Urinary and genitals	Urologist	_____
Tumors and treatment	Oncologist	_____
Ear, nose, throat, and voice box	Otorhino-laryngologist	_____

88.

Here are 42 more medical terms you have worked with in Unit 9. Don't forget to pronounce each one carefully before taking the final Unit 9 Self-test.

apnea (ap′ nē ə)

blepharedema (blef′ ar ə dē′ mä)

blepharoptosis (blef ar op tō′ sis)

bronchitis (brong kī′ tis)

bronchoscopy (brong kos′ kō pē)

corectopia (kōr ek tō′ pē ə)

coreometer (kōr ē om′ e ter)

coreoplasty (kōr′ ē ō plas tē)

corneal (kor′ nē al)

cycloplegia (sī klō plē′ jē ə)

diplopia (di plō′ pē ə)

epistaxis (ep i stak′ sis)

hematemesis (hē mä tem′ ə sis)

hemoptysis (hē mop′ ti sis)

iridocele (ir id ō sēl)

iridoplegia (ir id ō plē′ jē ə)

iritis (ī rī′ tis)

keratome (ker′ ə tōm)

keratoplasty (ker′ ə tō plas tē)

keratoscleritis (ker′ ə tō skler ī′ tis)

keratotomy (ker a tōt′ ō mē)

laryngeal (la rin′ jē al)

laryngospasm (la ring′ gō spazm)

nasolacrimal (nā zō lak′ ri məl)

nasomental (nā zō men′ təl)

nasopharyngitis (nā′ zō fair in jī′ tis)

ophthalmoscope (of thal′ mō skōp)

pharyngitis (fair in jī′ tis)

pharyngotomy (fair in got′ ō mē)

pleuralgia (plōō ral′ jē ə)

pleurisy (plōōr′ i sē)

pleurocentesis (plōōr′ ō sen tē′ sis)

pneumohemothorax (nyōō mō hē mō thōr′ aks)

pneumonia (nyōō mō′ nē ə)

retinitis (ret i nī′ tis)

retinoscopy (ret i nos′ kō pē)

sclerectomy (skler ek′ tō mē)

singultus (sing gul′ tus)

tracheorrhagia (trā kē ō rāj′ jē ə)

tracheostomy (trā kē os′ tō mē)

thorax (thor′ aks)

thoracocentesis (thôr′ ə kō sen tē′ sis)

Unit 9 Self-Test

PART 1

From the list on the right, select the correct meaning for each of the following often used medical terms.

_____ 1. Pneumonectomy

_____ 2. Keratoscleritis

_____ 3. Pleurocentesis

_____ 4. Corectasia

_____ 5. Pleuralgia

_____ 6. Blepharedema

_____ 7. Hemoptysis

_____ 8. Ophthalmologist

_____ 9. Nasomental

_____ 10. Iridoplegia

_____ 11. Tracheorrhagia

_____ 12. Keratome

_____ 13. Epistaxis

_____ 14. Retinoid

_____ 15. Bronchitis

a. Nosebleed

b. Spitting blood

c. Pertaining to nose and chin

d. Stretching (dilation) of the pupil

e. Puncture of the pleural space to remove fluid

f. Pain of the pleura

g. Instrument to cut the cornea

h. Paralysis of the iris

i. Inflammation of cornea and sclera

j. Resembling the retina

k. Swollen eyelids due to fluid in the tissues

l. Physician who specializes in the study of eye diseases

m. Hermorrhage from the trachea

n. Inflammation of the bronchi

o. Surgical removal of a lung

PART 2

Write the medical term for each of the following brief definitions.

1. Air in the chest   _____
2. Pertaining to nose and tears   _____
3. Incision into the throat   _____
4. Hiccup   _____
5. Instrument to examine the eye   _____
6. Plastic surgery of the cornea   _____
7. Double vision   _____
8. Drooping eyelid   _____
9. Pain in the covering of the lung   _____
10. Permanent opening into the
    windpipe   _____
11. Inflammation of the iris   _____
12. Spasm of the voice box   _____
13. Pertaining to the cornea   _____
14. Paralysis of the ciliary body   _____
15. Very fast breathing   _____

ANSWERS

Part 1

1. o	9. c
2. i	10. h
3. e	11. m
4. d	12. g
5. f	13. a
6. k	14. j
7. b	15. n
8. l	

Part 2

1. Pneumothorax	9. Pleurodynia
2. Nasolacrimal	10. Tracheostomy
3. Pharyngotomy	11. Iritis
4. Singultus	12. Laryngospasm
5. Ophthalmoscope	13. Corneal
6. Keratoplasty	14. Cycloplegia
7. Diplopia	15. Tachypnea
8. Blepharoptosis	

Review Sheets

Unit 1: Review Sheet

PART 1

WORD PART	MEANING	
acr/o-	_____	extremity
megal/o-	_____	enlargement
dermat/o-	_____	skin
cyan/o-	_____	blue
derm/o-	_____	skin
leuk/o-	_____	white
-itis	_____	inflammation
cardi/o-	_____	heart
gastr/o-	_____	stomach
cyt/o-	_____	cell
-ologist	_____	one who studies
-algia	_____	pain
-ectomy	_____	excision
-otomy	_____	incision
-ostomy	_____	new opening
duoden/o-	_____	duodenum
electr/o-	_____	electricity
-ology	_____	study of
-osis	_____	condition of
-tome	_____	instrument that cuts
gram/o-	_____	record
eti/o-	_____	cause of
path/o-	_____	disease

PART 2

MEANING	WORD PART	
record	_____	gram/o-
one who studies (suffix)	_____	-ologist
enlargement	_____	megal/o-
electricity	_____	electr/o-
white	_____	leuk/o-
incision (suffix)	_____	-otomy
blue	_____	cyan/o-
instrument that cuts (suffix)	_____	-tome
stomach	_____	gastr/o-
extremity	_____	acr/o-
condition of (suffix)	_____	-osis
disease	_____	path/o-
new opening (suffix)	_____	-ostomy
skin	_____	dermat/o-, derm/o-
study of (suffix)	_____	-ology
heart	_____	cardi/o-
excision (suffix)	_____	-ectomy
inflammation (suffix)	_____	-itis
duodenum	_____	duoden/o-
pain (suffix)	_____	-algia
cell	_____	cyt/o-
cause of	_____	eti/o-

Unit 2: Review Sheet

PART 1

WORD PART	MEANING	
aden/o-	_____	gland
carcin/o-	_____	cancer
malac/o-	_____	soft, softened
-oid	_____	resembling
laryng/o-	_____	larynx
cephal/o-	_____	head
hyper-	_____	excessive, more than normal
-cele	_____	herniation
ost/o-, oste/o-	_____	bone
arthr/o-	_____	joint
chondr/o-	_____	cartilage
cost/o-	_____	rib
lip/o-	_____	fat
inter-	_____	between
dent/o-	_____	tooth
-emesis	_____	vomiting
-oma	_____	tumor
-plast/o, -plast/y	_____	repair
hypo-	_____	under, less than normal
troph/o-	_____	development
morph/o-	_____	structure and form
muc/o-	_____	mucus
onc/o-	_____	tumor
hist/o-	_____	tissue(s)
en-, endo-	_____	inside, within
ex-, exo-	_____	out, completely outside

PART 2

MEANING	WORD PART	
rib	_____	cost/o-
larynx	_____	laryng/o-
development	_____	troph/o-
cancer	_____	carcin/o-
repair (suffix)	_____	-plast/o(/y)
tooth	_____	dent/o-
mucus	_____	muc/o-
under, less than normal	_____	hypo-
herniation (suffix)	_____	-cele
soft, softened	_____	malac/o-
gland	_____	aden/o-
tumor (suffix)	_____	-oma
bone	_____	oste/o-
vomiting (suffix)	_____	-emesis
head	_____	cephal/o-
joint	_____	arthr/o-
between (prefix)	_____	inter-
resembling (suffix)	_____	-oid
fat	_____	lip/o-
inside, within (prefix)	_____	en-, endo-
cartilage	_____	chondr/o-
excessive, more than normal (prefix)	_____	hyper-
tissue	_____	hist/o-
structure and form	_____	morph/o-
tumor(s)	_____	onc/o-
out, completely outside (prefix)	_____	ex-, exo-

Unit 3: Review Sheet

PART 1

WORD PART	MEANING	
cyst/o-	_____	bladder
-ar	_____	pertaining to
crani/o-	_____	cranium (skull)
dipl/o-	_____	double
cerebr/o-	_____	cerebrum
ab-	_____	away from
cocc/i-	_____	coccus
metr/o-meter-	_____	measure
py/o-	_____	pus
-genesis, gen/o-	_____	produce, originate
-orrhea	_____	flow
ot/o-	_____	ear
-centesis	_____	puncture
rhin/o-	_____	nose
lith/o-	_____	stone or calculus
hydr/o-	_____	water
chol/e-	_____	gall, bile
thorac/o-	_____	thorax or chest
pelv/i-	_____	pelvis
ad-	_____	toward
abdomin/o-	_____	abdomen
therap/o-	_____	treatment
lumbo-	_____	loin
phob/ia	_____	fear
supra-	_____	above

PART 2

MEANING	WORD PART
water	_____ hydr/o-
flow (suffix)	_____ -orrhea
fear	_____ phob/ia
double	_____ dipl/o-
loin	_____ lumb/o-
pelvis	_____ pelv/i-
gall, bile	_____ chol/e-
nose	_____ rhin/o-
puncture (suffix)	_____ -centesis
cerebrum	_____ cerebr/o-
pus	_____ py/o-
treatment	_____ therap/o-
toward (prefix)	_____ ad-
produce, originate (suffix), (prefix)	_____ -genesis, gen/o-
above (prefix)	_____ supra-
bladder	_____ cyst/o-
coccus	_____ cocc/i-
measure	_____ metr/o-, meter-
stone or calculus	_____ lith/o-
ear	_____ ot/o-
thorax or chest	_____ thorac/o-
cranium (skull)	_____ crani/o-
away from (prefix)	_____ ab-
abdomen	_____ abdomin/o-
above (prefix)	_____ supra-

Unit 4: Review Sheet

PART 1

WORD/WORD PART	MEANING	
-peps/ia	_____	digestion
neur/o-	_____	nerve
blast/o-	_____	embryonic form
a-, an-	_____	without
angi/o-	_____	vessel
-spasm	_____	twitching
scler/o-	_____	hard
-tachy	_____	fast
aneurysm	_____	ballooning-out vessel
fibr/o-	_____	fibrous, fiber
lys/o-	_____	destruction, dissolution
pne/o-	_____	breathe
arteri/o-	_____	artery
men/o-	_____	menses
hemat/o-, hemo-	_____	blood
kinesi/o-	_____	movement
spermat/o-	_____	spermatozoon
oophor/o-, o-o-	_____	ovary
-pexy	_____	fixation
salping/o-	_____	fallopian tube
dys-	_____	bad, painful, difficult
hyster/o-	_____	uterus
-ptosis	_____	prolapse, drooping
-brady	_____	slow
anomaly	_____	irregularity, breaks the rule
ur/o-	_____	urine
nephr/o-	_____	kidney
pyel/o-	_____	renal pelvis
ureter/o-	_____	ureter
-orrhaphy	_____	suture

urethr/o-   _____   urethra
-orrhagia   _____   hemorrhage
colp/o-   _____   vagina
crypt/o-   _____   hidden
pne/o-   _____   breathing
orchid/o-   _____   testis
hernia   _____   protrusion
                                                        through cavity
                                                        wall

PART 2

MEANING   WORD/WORD PART

artery   _____   arteri/o-
vessel   _____   angi/o-
uterus   _____   hyster/o-
movement   _____   kinesi/o-
destruction,
    dissolution   _____   lys/o-
blood   _____   hemat/o-,
                                                        hem/o-

protrusion through
    cavity wall   _____   hernia
urine   _____   ur/o-
hard   _____   scler/o-
slow (prefix)   _____   brady-
fallopian tube   _____   salping/o-
muscle   _____   my/o-
without (prefix) _____   a-, an-
nerve   _____   neur/o-
fixation (suffix) _____   -pexy
embryonic form   _____   blast/o-
ballooning-out
    vessel   _____   aneurysm
ovary   _____   oophor/o-, o-o-
breathe   _____   pne/o-
digestion   _____   -peps/ia
prolapse, drooping _____   -ptosis
bad, painful,
    difficult (prefix) _____   dys-
spermatozoa   _____   spermat/o-

fibrous, fiber	_____	fibr/o-
twitching (suffix)	_____	-spasm
fast (suffix)	_____	-tachy
hemorrhage (suffix)	_____	-orrhagia
renal pelvis	_____	pyel/o-
vagina	_____	colp/o-
ureter	_____	ureter/o-
kidney	_____	nephr/o-
irregularity, breaks the rule	_____	anomaly
urethra	_____	urethr/o-
suture (suffix)	_____	-orrhaphy
hidden	_____	crypt/o-
testes	_____	orchid/o-
menses	_____	men/o-

Unit 5: Review Sheet

PART 1

WORD/WORD PART	MEANING	
stomat/o-	_____	mouth
gloss/o-	_____	tongue
cheil/o-	_____	lips
gingiv/o-	_____	gums
esophag/o-	_____	esophagus
enter/o-	_____	small intestine
thrombus	_____	blood clot
col/o-	_____	colon
rect/o-	_____	rectum
proct/o-	_____	anus or rectum
hepat/o-	_____	liver
pancreat/o-	_____	pancreas
clys/o-, -clys/is	_____	wash, irrigate
-ectasia	_____	dilatation, stretched
-pleg/a (/ia, /ic)	_____	paralysis
phleb/o-	_____	vein
dys-	_____	bad, difficult, painful
-orrhexis	_____	rupture
esthesia	_____	feeling, sensation
fibrillation	_____	very fast heartbeat
algesia	_____	of pain sensation
phas/o-	_____	speech
-scope, -scopy	_____	look, examine
-tripsy	_____	surgical crushing
plas/o-	_____	formation, development
syn-sym-	_____	together as one
splen/o-	_____	spleen
embolus	_____	foreign particle in the blood
dactyl/o-	_____	fingers, toes

macro-	_____	large
embolism	_____	vessel blocked by an embolus
myel/o-	_____	spinal cord, bone marrow
poly-	_____	many
jejun/o-	_____	jejunum
micro-	_____	very small
ile/o	_____	ileum
defibrillation	_____	restoration of regular heartbeat (usually with electric shock)

PART 2

MEANING	WORD/WORD PART	
paralysis (suffix)	_____	-pleg/a (/ia, /ic)
liver	_____	hepat/o-
blood clot	_____	thrombus
small intestine	_____	enter/o-
feeling, sensation	_____	esthesia
speech	_____	phas/o-
sensation of pain	_____	algesia
anus or rectum	_____	proct/o-
lips	_____	cheil/o-
wash, irrigate (suffix)	_____	-clys/o-, -clys/is
esophagus	_____	esophag/o-
colon	_____	col/o-
gums	_____	gingiv/o-
mouth	_____	stomat/o-
vein	_____	phleb/o-
dilatation, stretched (suffix)	_____	-ectasia
pancreas	_____	pancreat/o
rectum	_____	rect/o-
tongue	_____	gloss/o-
vessel blocked by an embolus	_____	embolism

restoration of regular heartbeat (usually with electric shock)	_____	defibrillation
foreign particle in the blood	_____	embolus
formation, development	_____	plas/o-
rupture (suffix)	_____	-orrhexis
bad, difficult, painful (prefix)	_____	dys-
surgical crushing (suffix)	_____	-trips/y
ileum	_____	ile/o-
jejunum	_____	jejun/o-
look, examine (suffix)	_____	-scope, -scopy
very small	_____	micr/o
large	_____	macr/o
bone marrow, spinal cord	_____	myel/o
finger or toe	_____	dactyl/o
many (prefix)	_____	poly-
with, together as one (prefix)	_____	syn-, sym-
very fast heartbeat	_____	fibrillation
spleen	_____	splen/o

Unit 6: Review Sheet

PART 1

WORD/WORD PART	MEANING	
edema	_____	fluid in the tissues
chronic	_____	long, drawn-out disease
syndrome	_____	symptoms occur together
prognosis	_____	prediction of course and outcome of disease
acute	_____	pertaining to severe symptom, rapid onset, short course
paroxysmal	_____	pertaining to sudden periodic attack
diagnosis	_____	identification of disease
tinnitus	_____	ringing in the ear
malaise	_____	vague sensation of not feeling well
vertigo	_____	sensation of turning around in space
anorexia	_____	loss of appetite
symptom	_____	perceived change in body or functions
pyrexia	_____	feverishness

mortality   _____   pertaining to being mortal

morbidity   _____   pertaining to being diseased

hypertrophy   _____   over-development

atrophy   _____   wasting away, shrinking of an organ

systemic   _____   pertaining to the whole body, all systems

vital signs   _____   T, P, and R

peripheral   _____   pertaining to the outside surface of the body

chlor/o-   _____   green

melan/o-   _____   black

erythr/o-   _____   red

xanth/o-   _____   yellow

prophylactic   _____   pertaining to prevention of disease

prodromal   _____   pertaining to phase of disease before symptoms

nausea   _____   seasickness, inclined to vomit

palliative   _____   pertaining to relief of symptoms, not cure

against (prefix)   _____   anti-

dyspnea   _____   difficult, painful breathing

hypothermia   _____   subnormal temperature, below 90°F

PART 2

MEANING	WORD/WORD PART	
symptoms occur together	_____	syndrome
prediction of course and outcome of disease	_____	prognosis
pertaining to severe symptom, rapid onset, short course	_____	acute
wasting away, shrinking of an organ	_____	atrophy
pertaining to the whole body, all systems	_____	systemic
T, P, and R	_____	vital signs
fluid in the tissues	_____	edema
long, drawn-out disease	_____	chronic
pertaining to sudden periodic attack	_____	paroxysmal
identification of disease	_____	diagnosis
ringing in the ear	_____	tinnitus
vague sensation of not feeling well	_____	malaise
sensation of turning around in space	_____	vertigo
loss of appetite	_____	anorexia
perceived change in body or functions	_____	symptom
pertaining to being diseased	_____	morbidity
pertaining to relief of symptoms, not cure	_____	palliative

fever	_____	pyret/o-, pyrexia
pertaining to phase of disease before symptoms	_____	prodromal
pertaining to prevention of disease	_____	prophylactic
yellow	_____	xanth/o-
red	_____	erythr/o-
seasickness, inclined to vomit	_____	nausea
black	_____	melan/o-
green	_____	chlor/o-
pertaining to the outside surface of the body	_____	peripheral
breathing reaches a climax, then ceases before starting again	_____	Cheyne-Stokes respiration
difficult, painful breathing	_____	dyspnea
overdevelopment	_____	hypertrophy
pertaining to being mortal	_____	mortality
feverishness	_____	pyret/o-, pyrexia
loss of appetite	_____	anorexia
symptoms occurring before the onset of the disease	_____	prodrome

Unit 7: Review Sheet

PART 1

WORD/WORD PART	MEANING	
supra-, super-	_____	above, over
cyst	_____	closed sac containing fluid
neoplasm	_____	new tissue growth, no purpose
lesion	_____	unhealthy, diseased tissue
infra-	_____	below, beneath, under
ectopic	_____	outside the normal place
ect/o-	_____	outside
papule, papula	_____	raised red spot, pimple
peri-	_____	around, about, nearby
ventral	_____	on or near the belly
epi-	_____	over, upon, surrounding
distal	_____	point farthest from trunk
dorsal	_____	on or near the back
epigastric	_____	area of the belly over the stomach
proximal	_____	point nearest to the trunk
papilloma	_____	nipple-shaped tumor on skin

lateral _____ farther from the midline

infiltration _____ slipping into and between normal cells

sub-, hypo- _____ below, beneath

excrescence _____ outgrowth, wart

medial _____ nearer to the midline

papilla _____ small, nipple-like protuberance

condyloma _____ perianal wartlike growth

benign _____ not spreading, not malignant

end/o- _____ inner, inside

malignant _____ bad kind, threatening death

tumor _____ new, abnormal tissue growth

metastasis _____ cells spread to new location

polyp _____ tumor on a little foot

circumscribed _____ as a line drawn around, edge

mes/o- _____ middle

PART 2

MEANING	WORD/WORD PART	
new, abnormal tissue growth	_____	tumor
cells spread to new location	_____	metastasis
middle (prefix)	_____	mes/o-
point nearest to the trunk	_____	proximal
perianal wartlike growth	_____	condyloma
not spreading, not malignant	_____	benign
inner, inside (prefix)	_____	end/o-
bad kind, threatening death	_____	malignant
closed sac containing fluid	_____	cyst
as a line drawn around, edge	_____	circumscribed
area of the belly over the stomach	_____	epigastric
new tissue growth, no purpose	_____	neoplasm
unhealthy, diseased tissue	_____	lesion
beneath the patella	_____	subpatellar, infrapatellar
outside the normal place	_____	ectopic
raised red spot, pimple	_____	papule, papula
around, circular (prefix)	_____	circum-
on or near the belly	_____	ventral
above the pubic arch	_____	suprapubic
below, beneath, under (prefix)	_____	infra-

on or near the back _____ dorsal

slipping into and
   between normal
   cells   _____ infiltration

tumor on a little
   foot   _____ polyp

over surrounding
   (prefix)   _____ epi-

around, about,
   nearby (prefix)   _____ peri-

under the skin   _____ hypodermic

point farthest from
   trunk   _____ distal

nipple-shaped
   tumor on skin   _____ papilloma

farther from the
   midline   _____ lateral

removal and
   examination
   of living tissue   _____ biopsy

Unit 8: Review Sheet

PART 1

WORD/WORD PART	MEANING	
conception	_____	union of ovum and spermatozoon
ovum	_____	female egg cell
peritoneum	_____	coats the viscera and lines the abdominal wall
secundi-	_____	second
fetus	_____	developing child in utero
spermatozoon	_____	male germ cell
parturition	_____	labor and delivery of term pregnancy
multi-	_____	many
nulli-	_____	none
postpartum	_____	after giving birth
mastopathy	_____	breast disease
hysterorrhexis	_____	rupture of uterus (life threatening)
metratrophy	_____	uterine atrophy
antepartum	_____	before labor
prenatal	_____	before childbirth
oligouria	_____	scanty urine formation
mamm/o-, mast/o	_____	breast
amniot/o-	_____	amnion (sac for fetus and fluid)
-atrophy	_____	wasting of an organ or part

primipara _____ a woman who
has given
birth for the
first time

-dynia _____ pain, painful

-mania _____ madness

-phobia _____ excessive fear

gravida _____ heavy with
child; a
pregnant
woman

men/o _____ menses,
menstruation

involution _____ process of uterus
returning to
nonpregnant
state

climacteric _____ change of life
period

placenta _____ organ that
nourishes
fetus in utero

gynecomastia _____ enlarged breasts
in a male

puerperium _____ period after
childbirth;
involution
takes place

pudenda _____ female external
genitals

gestation _____ another term for
pregnancy

amniocentesis _____ puncture of
amniotic sac
and removal
of fluid

perineum _____ pelvic floor;
region from
vulva to anus
in female

PART 2

MEANING	WORD/WORD PART
female external genitals	_____ pudenda
menses, menstruation	_____ men/o
madness (suffix)	_____ -mania
female egg cell	_____ ovum
wasting of an organ or part (suffix)	_____ -atrophy
another term for pregnancy	_____ gestation
puncture of amniotic sac and removal of fluid	_____ amniocentesis
enlarged breasts in a male	_____ gynecomastia
breast disease	_____ mastopathy
breast (word root)	_____ mast/o, mamm/o
none (prefix)	_____ nulli-
many (prefix)	_____ multi-
developing child in utero	_____ fetus
male germ cell	_____ spermatozoon
cessation of menses	_____ menopause
pregnant woman, first time	_____ primigravida
incision of vagina and pelvic outlet	_____ episiotomy
excessive fear (prefix)	_____ phobia-
pain, painful (suffix)	_____ -dynia
process of uterus returning to nonpregnant state	_____ involution
rupture of uterus (life threatening)	_____ hysterorrhexis

woman who has given birth	_____	para
pelvic floor; region from vulva to anus in female	_____	perineum
period after childbirth; involution takes place	_____	puerperium
amnion (sac for fetus and fluid) (word root)	_____	amniot/o
organ that nourishes fetus in utero	_____	placenta
few, little, scanty (prefix)	_____	oligo-
before labor	_____	antepartum
change of life period	_____	climacteric
physician specialist in diseases of women	_____	gynecologist
before (prefix)	_____	pre-
after (prefix)	_____	post-
new, recent (prefix)	_____	neo-
labor and delivery of term pregnancy	_____	parturition
X ray examination of breast	_____	mammography
coats viscera and abdominal wall	_____	peritoneum
union of ovum and spermatozoon	_____	conception
uterine atrophy	_____	metratrophy
pain, painful (suffix)	_____	-dynia
heavy with child; a pregnant woman	_____	gravida

Unit 9: Review Sheet

PART 1

WORD/WORD PART	MEANING
nas/o-	_____ nose
blephar/o-	_____ eyelid
scler/o-	_____ hard white coat of the eye
pharyng/o-	_____ pharynx, throat
ir, irid/o-	_____ iris, donut-shaped color of the eye
dipl/o-	_____ double, paired
laryng/o	_____ larynx, voice box
pneumon/o-	_____ lung
bronch/o-	_____ bronchus(i), branches of the trachea
ophthalm/o-	_____ eye
retin/o-	_____ retina, complex membrane on the inside back surface of the eyeball
pleur/o-	_____ pleura, covering on the lungs
core-, core/o-	_____ pupil, circular opening in the center of the eye
pne/o-	_____ breathing, breathe
lacrim/o-	_____ tear, tears
ment/o-	_____ chin
kerat/o-, corne/o-	_____ cornea, transparent covering of anterior one-sixth of the eye

thorac/o-	_____	thorax, chest
cycl/o-	_____	ciliary body, controls the shape of the iris
pneum/o-	_____	air, gases
trache/o-	_____	windpipe, trachea
singultus	_____	hiccup, hiccough
hemoptysis	_____	spitting of blood derived from the lungs
diaphragm	_____	musculo-membranous wall separating the abdomen from the thorax
epistaxis	_____	nosebleed

PART 2

MEANING	WORD/WORD PART	
nose	_____	nas/o-
breathing, breathe	_____	pne/o-
iris	_____	ir, irid/o-
larynx, voice box	_____	laryng/o-
cornea, transparent anterior covering of one-sixth of the eye	_____	kerat/o-, corne/o-
nosebleed	_____	epistaxis
spitting blood derived from the lungs	_____	hemoptysis

musculo-
   membranous
   wall separating
   the abdomen
   from the thorax   _____   diaphragm
air, gases   _____   pneum/o-
retina, complex
   membrane on
   the inside back
   surface of the
   eyeball   _____   retin/o-
pleura, covering on
   the lungs   _____   pleur/o-
eyelid   _____   blephar/o-
tear, tears   _____   lacrim/o-
windpipe, trachea   _____   trache/o-
pupil, circular
   opening in the
   center of the eye _____   core-, core/o-
hard white coat of
   the eye   _____   scler/o-
pharynx, throat   _____   pharyng/o-
bronchus(i),
   branches of the
   trachea   _____   bronch/o-
lung   _____   pneumon/o-
ciliary body,
   controls shape
   of the iris   _____   cycl/o-
thorax, chest   _____   thorac/o-
chin   _____   ment/o-
double, paired   _____   dipl/o-
eye   _____   ophthalm/o-
hiccup, hiccough   _____   singultus

Final Self-Test I

INSTRUCTIONS

INSTRUCTIONS

The following two tests will show you how much you have learned about medical terminology. Many of the words on the tests will be new to you; however, using the word parts and the word-building system you have learned, you should be able to give the meaning for all of them. Try these tests and see how well you do. You may want to take one test before reading the book and the other after you finish the book. The comparison will show even more clearly how much medical terminology you have learned.

Each test consists of 50 medical terms. For each term, write out a definition in your own words. Then compare your answers with those following the test. Your definition should include all of the ideas (though not necessarily in the exact words) as the definitions on the answer page.

TEST I

1. Tachypnea_____
2. Oophoritis _____
3. Pyelonephrosis_____
4. Pathogenic_____
5. Bradycardia_____
6. Cycloparalysis _____
7. Glossoplegia _____
8. Megalocardia _____
9. Ophthalmoscopy_____
10. Bronchopneumonogram _____
11. Mammopexy_____
12. Cystocele _____
13. Cephalometer _____
14. Herniorrhaphy _____

15. Hyperthyroidism _____
16. Bronchiectasis _____
17. Mastodynia _____
18. Xanthemia_____
19. Symptomatology _____
20. Etiology _____
21. Kinesialgia_____
22. Fibroosteoma _____
23. Anuria _____
24. Lipochondroma _____
25. Costectomy _____
26. Metastasis _____
27. Metrorrhagia _____
28. Paranephritis _____
29. Blepharoptosis _____
30. Erythrocyte _____
31. Perianal _____
32. Endocarditis _____
33. Lymphadenoid_____
34. Thoracolumbar_____
35. Corneoiritis _____
36. Hysterorrhexis _____
37. Thrombogenesis_____
38. Hematemesis _____
39. Lithotripsy_____
40. Oligohydramnios_____
41. Prostatic hypertrophy_____
42. Hemoptysis_____
43. Dorsalgia _____
44. Endocranial_____
45. Parturition_____
46. Adenocarcinoma _____
47. Esophagogastrostomy _____
48. Enterohepatitis_____
49. Malaise_____
50. Dyspnea_____

ANSWERS TO FINAL SELF-TEST I

1. rapid breathing
2. inflammation of an ovary
3. condition (abnormal or diseased) of the pelvis of the kidney
4. that which is capable of causing disease
5. slow heart rate
6. paralysis of the ciliary body
7. paralysis of the tongue
8. excessively large heart
9. examination of the interior of the eye
10. X ray of the bronchi and lungs
11. surgical fixation of a breast to its normal position
12. hernia of the bladder
13. instrument for measuring the head
14. suturing (repair) of a hernia
15. condition caused by excessive secretion of the thyroid glands
16. dilatation of the bronchi
17. painful breast
18. yellow pigment (color) in the blood
19. the study (science) of disease symptoms
20. the study of causes of disease
21. painful muscular movement
22. tumor of bone and fibrous connective tissue
23. absence of urine
24. tumor of cartilaginous and fatty tissue
25. excision of a rib or ribs
26. spreading of malignancy to another organ, location
27. uterine hemorrhage
28. inflammation of tissues around (surrounding) the kidney
29. drooping of an eyelid
30. red blood cell
31. of or pertaining to around the anus
32. inflammation of the inside (lining) of the heart
33. resembling a lymph gland
34. of or pertaining to the chest (thorax) and lower back (lumbar)
35. inflammation of the iris and cornea
36. rupture of the uterus
37. formation (development) of a clot (thrombus)
38. vomiting blood
39. crushing removal of a stone
40. scanty amniotic fluid
41. pertaining to enlargement of the prostate
42. spitting blood (from trachea, bronchi, or lungs)
43. pain in the back
44. of, or pertaining to, the inside of the head
45. labor and childbirth
46. malignant tumor of a gland
47. making a new opening (permanent) between the esophagus and the stomach
48. inflammation of the liver and intestine
49. vague sensation of not feeling well
50. difficult or painful breathing

Final Self-Test II

1. Mastoptosis _____
2. Epistaxis _____
3. Amenorrhea _____
4. Antipyretic _____
5. Nephrolith _____
6. Enterectasia _____
7. Paroxysmal _____
8. Encephalorrhagia _____
9. Craniocele _____
10. Anorexia _____
11. Gingivoglossitis _____
12. Cholecystitis _____
13. Abdominalgia _____
14. Arteriospasm _____
15. Adenosclerosis _____
16. Duodenohepatic _____
17. Endobronchoscopy _____
18. Iridoplegia _____
19. Tracheostomy _____
20. Megalogastria _____
21. Phleborrhexis _____
22. Cryptorchidism _____
23. Thromboid _____
24. Electroencephalogram _____
25. Hepatoma _____
26. Singultus _____
27. Intercostal _____
28. Epigastric _____
29. Urethrocystitis _____
30. Hypothyroidism _____
31. Traumatology _____
32. Pericardiectomy _____

33. Syndrome _____
34. Hepatorrhaphy _____
35. Megalodactylism _____
36. Nephropexy _____
37. Pneumonomelanosis _____
38. Cerebrovascular _____
39. Chondromalacia _____
40. Amniocentesis _____
41. Inframammary _____
42. Leukocytolysis _____
43. Salpingectomy _____
44. Hemodialysis _____
45. Metastasis _____
46. Xanthoderma _____
47. Ophthalmoplegia _____
48. Pneumohemothorax _____
49. Otorhinolaryngologist _____
50. Suprapubic _____

ANSWERS TO FINAL SELF-TEST II

1. pendulous, drooping breast
2. nosebleed
3. cessation of menstruation
4. a substance that counteracts (acts against) the effects of a fever
5. a stone (calculus) in the kidney
6. dilitation (stretching) of the small intestine
7. of, or pertaining to, a sudden recurrent onset of a condition (convulsions)
8. hemorrhage within the brain
9. hernia of structures in the skull (cranium)
10. loss of appetite
11. inflammation of the gums and tongue
12. inflammation of the gallbladder
13. painful abdomen
14. spasm (twitching) of an artery
15. condition of hardening of glandular tissue
16. of, or pertaining to, the duodenum and liver
17. examination of the inside of the bronchi
18. paralysis of the iris
19. making a new permanent opening in the trachea
20. excessively large stomach
21. rupture of a vein
22. condition due to hidden (undescended) testes
23. resembling a blood clot

24. record (picture) of electrical activity in the brain
25. tumor of the liver
26. hiccup, hiccough
27. between the ribs
28. of, or pertaining to, area of belly over stomach
29. inflammation of the urethra and bladder
30. condition of insufficient thyroid excretion
31. the study (science) of injuries and their effect on the body
32. excision of tissue around the heart
33. a group of symptoms occurring together
34. suturing (repairing) the liver
35. condition of abnormally large fingers and toes
36. surgical fixation of the kidney in its normal place
37. condition of black lungs, black lung disease
38. of, or pertaining to, the vessels of the brain
39. condition of softened cartilage tissue
40. puncture of the amniotic sac and withdrawing of fluid
41. below the breast
42. destruction of white blood cells
43. surgical removal of the fallopian tube
44. removal of toxic waste products from the blood
45. spreading of a malignant disease to another organ or location
46. skin of yellow color
47. paralysis of the eye
48. air and blood in the chest cavity
49. physician specialist in ear, nose, and voice box diseases
50. of, or pertaining to, the area above the pubis (pubic arch)

Appendix A:
Medical Abbreviations

ad libitum (ad. lib.)	As much as wanted; freely
ante cibum (a.c.)	Before meals
bis in die (b.i.d.)	Twice daily
(b.p.)	Blood pressure
cubic centimeter (cc.)	Cubic centimeter(s)
cum (/c)	With
en.	Enema
gram (g.)	Gram or grams
granum (gr.)	Grain or grains
gutta, guttae (gtt.)	Drop or drops
hoc nocte (h.n.)	Tonight
hora somni (h.s.)	At bedtime
l.	Liter(s)
oculus dexter (O.D.)	Right eye
oculus sinister (O.S.)	Left eye
oz.	Ounce
per anum (p.a.)	By, or through, the anus
per os (p.o.)	By, or through, the mouth
post cibum (p.c.)	After meals
pro re nata (p.r.n.)	According to circumstances
quaque die (q.d.)	Every day
quaque hora (q.h.)	Every hour
quater in die (q.i.d.)	Four times daily
signa (sig.)	Let it be labeled
sine (/s)	Without
statim (stat.)	Immediately; at once
suppositoria (suppos.)	Suppository
tabella (tab.)	Tablet
ter in die (t.i.d.)	Three times daily
T.	Temperature

Appendix B:
Forming Plurals

The following chart contains information about the formation of plurals from the singular form. Use it to work the frames that follow.

TO FORM PLURALS	
If the singular ending is	The plural ending is
a us um ma on is ix ex ax	ae (pronounce ae as ī) i a mata a es ices ⎫ ices ⎬ The word root is usually built aces ⎭ from the plural forms of words ending in ix, ex, and ax (e.g., radix, radic/es, radic/otomy, radic/i/form).

1.

bursae
bur´ sī   Form the plural of
conjunctivae   bursa _____;
kon junk´ tī vē   conjunctiva _____;
bacilli
bə sil´ ē   bacillus _____.

2.

vertebra
ver´ tə bra   Give the singular form of
nucleus   vertebrae _____;
nōō´ klē us   nuclei _____;
cornea
kor´ nē ə   cornea _____.

3.

atria

ā´ trē ə   Form the plural of

cocci   atrium _____;

kok´ sī   coccus _____;

ilea

(you pronounce)   ileum _____.

il´ ē ə

4.

enema   Give the singular form of

en´ ə mä   enemata _____;

bacterium   bacteria _____;

ovum   ova _____.

(you pronounce)

5.

cortices   Form the plural of

kor´ ti sēz   cortex _____;

fibromata

fī brō´ mä tä   fibroma _____;

protozoa

prō´ to zō´ ə   protozoon _____.

6.

stigma   Give the singular form of

stig´ mä   stigmata _____;

prognosis

prog nō´ sis   prognoses _____;

spermatozoon

sper mat´ ə zō ən   spermatozoa _____.

7.
Form the plural of

appendices
(you pronounce)
appendix _____;

diagnoses
dī ag nō′ sēz
diagnosis _____;

ganglia
gang′ lē ä
ganglion _____.

8.
Refer to the table. Give the word root that usually refers to

appendic
the appendix _____;

cortic
the cortex _____;

thorac
(you pronounce)
the thorax _____.

9.
With this new knowledge, which you found for yourself, build a word meaning inflammation of the appendix,

appendic/itis
a pen di sī′ tis
_____ / _____;

cortic/al
kor′ ti kəl
pertaining to the cortex,
_____ / _____;

thorac/o/centesis
thor′ ə kō sen tē′
   sis
surgical puncture of the thorax,
_____ / _____ / _____.

10.
Form the plural of

apices
apex _____;

fornices
fornex _____;

varices
varix _____;

sarcomata
sarcoma _____;

septa
septum _____;

radii
radius _____;

maxillae
(you pronounce)
maxilla _____.

11.
There are other ways of forming plurals. They apply to only a few words. When you meet these words and have a question about how their plural forms are built, consult a medical dictionary.

Index of Word Parts Learned

The following word parts are listed by page number.